Anatomy of an Injury

A Patients' Introduction to Rehabilitation

Rachel A. Feinberg, MD

Barry I. Feinberg, MD

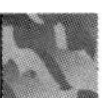

We must also express our thanks to Vicki Lander, Certified Massage Therapist. She has gifted hands, wisdom, a kind soul, and a positive and inspiring philosophy, and she puts into words an essential component that is often neglected in the rehabilitation process: the importance of self-care.

Sara Jenkins, our editor, worked hard to ensure that this book is clear and useful to readers. Her input was thoughtful and well worth the time and effort involved. Michael Reddy's ability to visualize the text is demonstrated in his fine illustrations, which facilitate readers' understanding of difficult concepts. The book was designed by Denise Gibson, whose enthusiasm and commitment resulted in a book that is not only handsome and readable but distinctive in its style.

Along with all this talent, one person was essential in bringing the book to completion: Joy Bush. Her meticulous organizational skills, her tireless typing and editing, her calm intelligence in overseeing a complex project, her faith, and above all her loyalty brought us all together to produce this book. She comforted our wounded spirits at moments of doubt and fatigue, and she kept us moving steadily toward the final goal.

To all these people we express our warmest appreciation.

Rachel and Barry Feinberg

CONTENTS

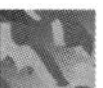

The members of our health care team—physicians, physical therapists, nurses, technicians, and administrative staff—feel an obligation to practice the traditional art of medicine while utilizing the extensive resources of modern science. Our approach to **rehabilitation** integrates injury anatomy, injury physiology, and injury structural and functional changes and their effects on pain. It also includes educating patients about the connection between pain and abnormal structure and function.

The four phases of treatment as practiced in our clinic are as follows:

- manual therapy, such as myofascial release, in conjunction with injection therapy to decrease pain and increase range of motion
- neuromuscular facilitation to correct abnormal movement patterns
- functional retraining: practicing correct movement patterns until they become habitual
- aerobic reconditioning (exercise such as walking, running, and cycling) to increase blood flow to muscles and connective tissues to maintain physiological well-being and reduce probability of re-injury.

Ongoing self-maintenance continues after formal rehabilitation, with individualized programs tailored to each patient's particular needs. These may include referrals to massage, yoga, and movement specialists in the community—not as an alternative but as an integral part of the rehabilitative process.

Unfortunately, we still do not know everything about the mechanisms in the nervous system that cause and inhibit pain. But by paying attention to detail in analyzing patient movement patterns, we can continually improve rehabilitative techniques. Physicians, therapists, and patients all can contribute to understanding the "anatomy of an injury."

rehabilitation: restoring normal functioning after injury or disease

PART I

ANATOMY OF AN INJURY

> *"Our nature consists of movement; absolute rest is death."*
>
> **Blaise Pascal, 1623–1662 *(Pensées)***

1 How Injury Happens

This book is about rehabilitation after **soft-tissue** injury, which is a common and greatly misunderstood source of **chronic** pain. The following chapters use the joint as a model for understanding a soft-tissue injury. A joint is made up of both hard tissue (bone) and soft tissue (muscle, tendon, ligament, cartilage, nerves, and connective tissue). Both hard and soft tissue are essential in maintaining the structural integrity and biomechanical function of the joint. Because soft tissues are extremely pain-sensitive, they can affect overall joint movement.

Understanding how an injury develops requires a knowledge of both the structure of the joint, or the anatomy, and its function, or biomechanics.

Signs and symptoms that constitute an injury are best understood by tracing the sequence of events leading up to it. Often these events start months before the first complaint of pain. In fact, if the affected joint were viewed through time-lapse photography, a sequence of abnormal structural and functional changes that ultimately resulted in injury would be revealed.

WHAT IS AN INJURY?

Trauma to a joint and/or muscle that moves the joint causes irritation and inflammation, which causes

soft tissue: muscles, tendons, ligaments, organs, connective tissue, skin, cartilage—everything but bones

chronic: continuing or recurring frequently over a long period

trauma: injury

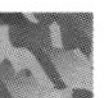

pain. The affected joint is not only painful but also will become **dysfunctional**. The cause of an injury can range from a single traumatic event to a series of repeated strains.

Understanding how an injury develops requires a knowledge of both the *structure* of the joint, or the anatomy, and its *function*, or biomechanics. With this knowledge, the dysfunction can be identified precisely. Only then can the correct diagnosis be made and a treatment plan designed. If the cause of the injury cannot be identified, the treatment plan will not be rational.

MOVEMENT

Movement of a joint requires two different types of input, the first of which is energy. In the body, energy comes from blood supply, as blood brings oxygen to the tissues. When blood supply is inadequate, fatigue develops. Then a joint is not able to move efficiently, and dysfunction results.

Movement also requires "information" from the nerves, or neural input, so that the actions involved occur in the proper sequence. Neural input is basically **imprinted**; we don't control it. An axiom in physical therapy states that the brain knows nothing of individual muscle action, only of movement. For example, when the knee bends, we do not consciously think, "First, tighten the hamstring muscle, then relax the quadriceps muscle," but, simply, "I am going to bend my knee." However, if you just got out of bed feeling stiff and sore after a day of hard exercise, you may not bend your knee in the same carefree way as when you are symptom-free. You may consciously decide to move slowly and carefully. Thus, the sequence of actions in a movement is dependent upon subconscious neural input but can be overridden by conscious thought.

dysfunctional: unable to function normally

imprinting: patterns of learned responses established early in life

When injury occurs, either from inadequate blood supply or from a change in neural input, a dysfunctional pattern develops. To compensate for the functional loss caused by the injury, we repeat the pattern, which causes further problems that eventually can lead to chronic pain. A muscle has a primary, secondary, and tertiary action. When injured, a muscle cannot efficiently perform its primary action and recruits an associated muscle. This cascade of **compensation** leads to dysfunction and repetitive strain because the recruited muscle will not be available to perform its primary action. For example, if the knee is stiff, causing a limp, the back and hip muscles may be recruited to make gait possible. Eventually, the back, hip, and knee will become painful and dysfunctional.

When injury occurs, a dysfunctional pattern develops. To compensate for the dysfunction, we repeat the pattern, which causes further problems that can lead to chronic pain.

The central nervous system is made up of the brain and spinal cord (Fig. 1-1A). Neural information comes from the periphery of the body (Fig. 1-1B)—arms, legs, or torso—and is processed by the central nervous system. Information may include pain, absence of pain, numbness, temperature, and position sense (i.e., where the body part is in space). Information is processed in the central nervous system through complicated neural pathways. This may lead to conscious as well as subconscious movement. For example, nerves going out from the spinal cord send information directly to the muscles, causing them to contract (shorten), which results in the desired movement (Fig. 1-2). Which muscles contract to create movement, and in what order, is the key to how a repetitive injury develops. The sequence of contractions is subconscious.

Neural information follows a particular path in the body. For example, from the nerve receptors in a finger, a pain impulse travels through **afferent**

compensation: using another muscle instead of one that is injured

afferent: nerves carrying impulses from the periphery of the body to the central nervous system

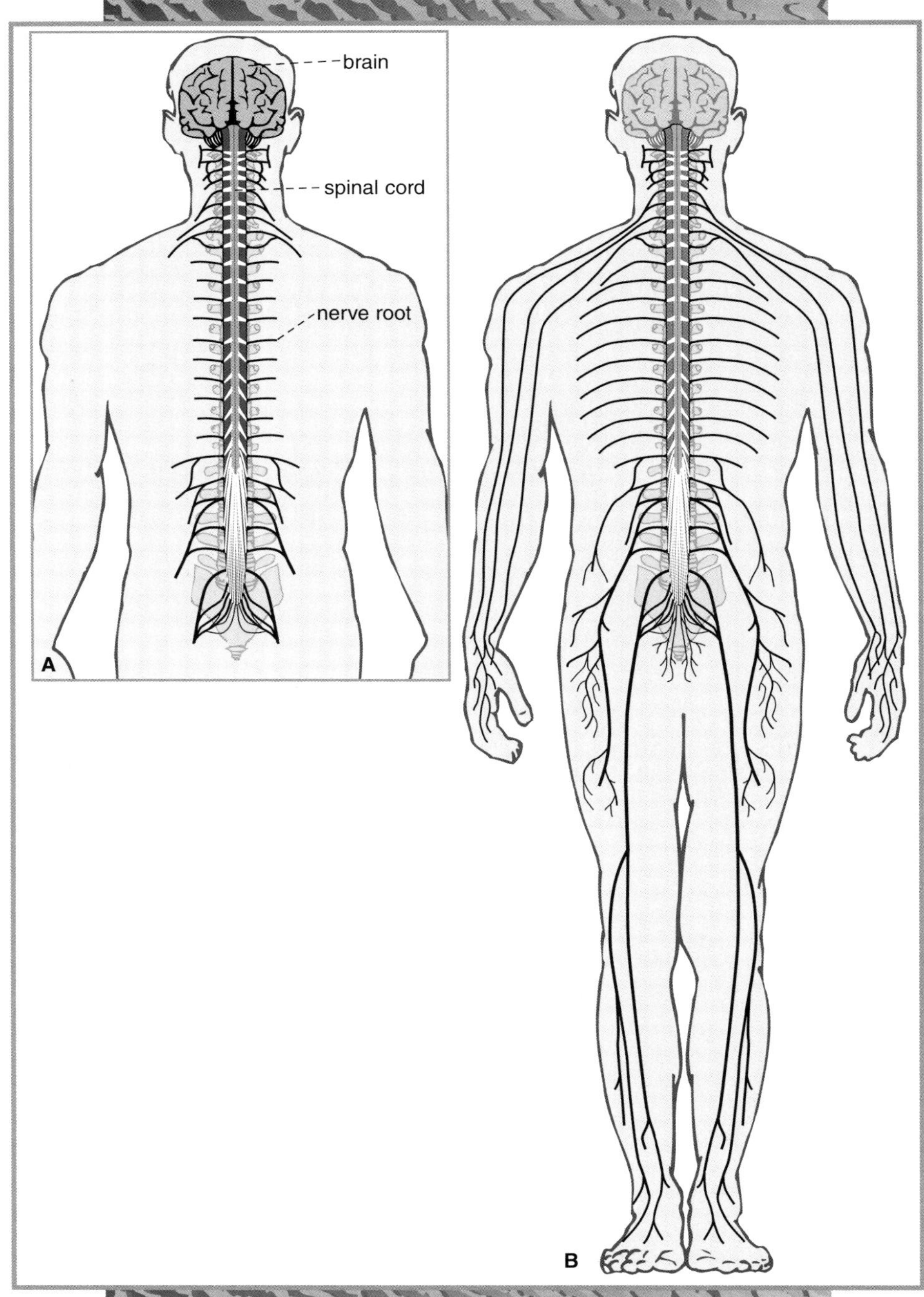

FIG. 1-1. Nervous system. A) Central. B) Peripheral.

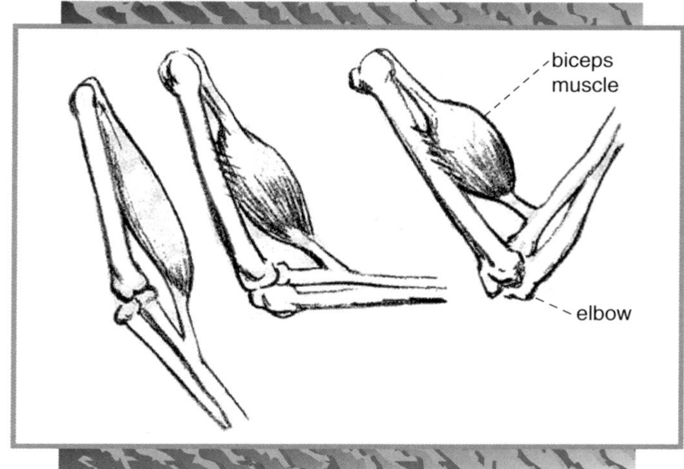

FIG. 1-2. Muscle contraction resulting in movement of a joint.

nerves to the central nervous system where it is processed. Information may then return via **efferent** nerves to produce a response (Fig. 1-3).

A joint requires specific anatomical alignment to allow proper movement. Abnormal posture increases stress in a particular joint. If you stand with your head forward or your back swayed, or if you work constantly stooped over, you are placing the joint at a mechanical disadvantage, thus making the joint accommodate movement from an abnormal position. This is similar to driving a car through difficult terrain on a daily basis. The constant stress will affect the car's mechanical condition, and the car's performance will suffer, with increased wear and decreased efficiency in fuel consumption. Similarly, improper posture increases stress and energy demands in the joints. If enough energy (blood supply) is not provided to the joint, another joint or muscle group may overwork to compensate.

A joint requires specific anatomical alignment to allow proper movement.

Chronic soft-tissue injury results in a loss of water in the tissue, which translates into loss of elasticity. This loss of elasticity causes deformation of support structures when they are placed under mechanical load. The muscles also lose **range of motion** and flexibility. When muscles stiffen, they develop trigger points ("charlie horses"), which are painful areas of partially contracted muscle. Such muscles are subject

efferent: nerves carrying impulses outward from the central nervous system

range of motion: full extent to which a joint can move

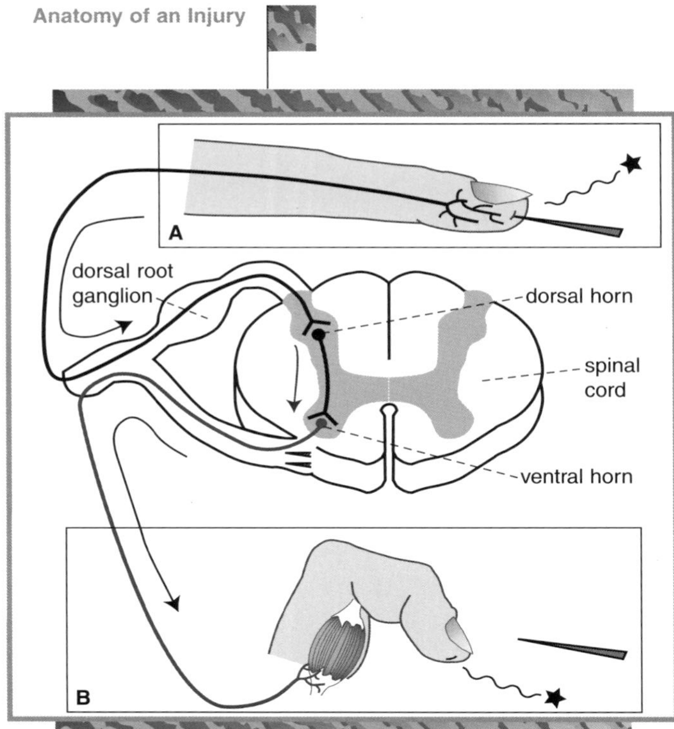

FIG. 1-3. Finger exposed to painful stimulus and processing of neural information, shown through cross section of spinal cord. A) Injury: pain impulse travels to central nervous system. B) Information from central nervous system causes withdrawal of finger.

to fatigue. Poor circulation results, and eventually inflammation and scarring occur. As the muscles and joints scar, the nerves can become trapped, and free motion of the nerve is impeded. Part of the rehabilitative process is to relieve the tension on the neural component.

Movement of a joint requires **neuromuscular coordination**, or proper sequencing of actions. An injury disrupts this sequence; pain and dysfunction alter coordinated movement as the body tries to determine the least painful way to move. But the least painful way may not be the proper way to move. Each particular movement of a joint generally requires a coordinated action of three to eight muscles. The body allows only a limited deviation from normal anatomy and motion patterns without dysfunctional consequences. Repetition and learning of these patterns leads to neural imprinting. When a young person falls, pain or dysfunction may develop, but because young muscle is more elastic, the injury may heal before dysfunction occurs. With age, our blood supply, muscle elasticity, and neuromuscular

neuromuscular coordination: normal pattern of nerves and muscles working together

coordination become limited, and there is less capacity to recover quickly from injury.

EFFECTS OF STRESS AND STRAIN

If an abnormal movement pattern develops, the result is a dysfunctional motion, which leads to easy fatigue, compensation, pain, and stiffness.

Joint motion requires muscle contraction. As the work load of a joint increases through continued movement or increased resistance, the contracting muscle will engage more of its fibers to accomplish the task (see Fig. 1-2). As demands increase beyond the muscle's ability to use more fibers, the body compensates by recruiting additional muscles which may result in motion of other joints. For example, to lift a paper from the floor, a simple contraction of the biceps muscle is enough. To lift a box of paper, you need to recruit all the fibers of your biceps. However, to lift a crate of paper, the biceps alone are not strong enough, so you might need to use more muscles in your arms and even bend your legs so that other muscles can help. Similarly, a relatively simple task repeated frequently in a short period of time can exhaust the available energy supply to the joints and muscles involved. In such cases, the body will make compensations to attempt to perform a task in the most energy-efficient and pain-free manner.

The autonomic nervous system acts as a computer designed to efficiently regulate blood flow and energy. When the pattern of joint motion is changed by injury or stress—for example, in the way we throw a ball—the information encoded in the nervous system that determines this motion is changed as well. We may then throw the ball awkwardly, adding further strain to the joint. The joint motion is then retrained in the new, altered movement pattern. Repeating the pattern over and

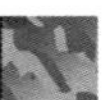

over (practice) makes the movement automatic. Eventually, the new pattern is recognized as "normal" and is reflexively (automatically) performed. If an abnormal movement pattern develops, the result is a dysfunctional motion, which leads to easy fatigue, compensation, pain, and stiffness. When compensation is no longer possible, further deviation from the correct movement pattern causes pain with all movement of the joint.

Immobilization relays a message to the central nervous system that energy is not currently needed in that joint. Therefore, blood flow is shunted away from immobile joints to active body parts. When the injured joint is forced to move, the pain intensifies. The pain also spreads; pain that began in the wrist may be felt in the entire arm. The shoulder joint may begin to move incorrectly to compensate for the initially painful wrist joint. Thus, pain and dysfunction spread from the site of the initial injury. Furthermore, the reduced blood flow creates an unhealthy, energy-poor environment for muscle, which perpetuates the cycle of dysfunction and pain.

Injury ➡ Change in alignment ➡ Dysfunctional movement ➡ Pain ➡ Spread of pain

The nerve branches are placed under tension at the level of the dysfunctional joint, which can immobilize the nerve throughout its entire length.

For example, many injuries begin just this simply: someone working on a production line may perform the same motion over and over again inappropriately. The worker feels stiffness and pain in the wrist but continues working. When the pain progresses, he or she visits a physician. The physician takes an x-ray which shows that the joint appears to be normal. The worker returns to the same job. The pain spreads. By the time the pain is re-evaluated, the entire arm and shoulder hurt, and eventually the shoulder becomes immobile. This is why the functional process needs to be evaluated early, and proper diagnosis is critical. As the nerves pass stressed joints and/or muscles, they can become compressed. This causes changes that can be detected by electromyography and nerve conduction velocity testing (see Chapter 5).

Physical conditioning—training to improve physical performance—increases the capacity for motion without fatigue. Practicing a correct movement pattern with a joint or muscle group works therapeutically to retrain the body and increase force and speed, in the same way that athletes do in their training. Once an athlete learns a motion properly, conditioning enables maximum performance of that motion. The same approach is used in rehabilitation. Conditioning improves blood supply, and increased blood supply (which provides energy) prevents fatigue. In that way, normal motion reduces problems for the body.

Practicing a correct movement pattern with a joint or muscle group works therapeutically to retrain the body and increase force and speed, in the same way that athletes do in their training.

Normal structure and function are also affected by nutrition. Obesity, in addition to decreasing blood flow to joints, increases the shear and compressive forces in the joints. Such constant stresses eventually alter normal structure and function. Poor nutrition also may cause anemia, which, like smoking, can lead to decreased oxygen supply to muscles and joint tissues. Also, muscle mass is dependent upon adequate protein intake, and excessive alcohol consumption is extremely harmful to protein metabolism. While alcohol may temporarily blunt pain, in the long run pain is intensified as alcohol depletes the body's own pain-relieving hormones. An individual who drinks, smokes, and is overweight and poorly conditioned is more prone to developing an injury and certainly faces a more prolonged recovery.

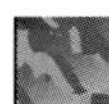

Previous injuries or scar tissue from surgical procedures also may affect the development of an injury and the rehabilitation process. Scars from a surgical incision may involve all layers of tissue from the skin to the joint itself. The changes in anatomy as a result of surgery or a pre-existing injury can lead to dysfunctional movement and ultimately an abnormal pattern of joint motion. Permanent defects from severe injuries and congenital abnormalities may limit recovery. Therefore, the rehabilitation specialist needs to maximally correct anatomical abnormalities prior to retraining an injured joint to achieve the best possible outcome.

CONCLUSION

Pain and disability arise when stress and inflammation are greater than the body's ability to rest and repair the affected tissues. The healthier the person, the better their blood supply. The better the neuromuscular coordination, the more available are the protective mechanisms that prevent injury.

2 Anatomy and Pain

A common bias is that most pain comes from direct pressure on a spinal nerve root (called radicular pain, as in the familiar example of a herniated disc). This assumption is made not only by patients but by physicians, attorneys, and insurance companies. For example, it often happens in the course of a day at the clinic that a patient walks in and insists on having an MRI or a CT scan, believing that his or her intense arm, leg, or back pain is caused by a herniated disc and that a sophisticated and expensive scan is the first step toward solving the problem.

Pain is a symptom of inflammation and irritation, which can be caused by abnormal neural anatomy, abnormal movement, abnormal position, or all three.

We are faced with trying to teach, as we explained in Chapter 1, that pain is often a symptom of inflammation and irritation. It can be caused by pathologic neural anatomy, abnormal movement, abnormal position, or all three. In our experience, a great deal of pain is actually caused by indirect tension on the nervous system as well as by direct nerve compression. It is this indirect tension that is often overlooked and misunderstood.

The aim of this chapter is to present a simplified explanation of the anatomic structures involved in the perception of pain. The mechanisms of pain are among the more complex topics in medicine. The

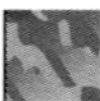

nervous system is made up of nerve cells that are elaborately interlaced. As described in Chapter 1, the nervous system consists of two divisions: the central nervous system is the brain and spinal cord, and the peripheral nervous system includes all other neural elements (nerve roots and sensory and motor nerves as well as the autonomic nervous system, described below). The nervous system as a whole regulates physical responses, both conscious and automatic, to the body's environment.

For sake of this discussion, the names of specific neural pathways in the brain and spinal cord are not important. But it is important to understand that painful stimuli from an injured site are transmitted through the nervous system from the periphery of the body to the spinal cord and brain, then modulated to either increase or decrease a patient's response to pain. Treatment is based on identifying the source of the pain within the pain pathway and then designing a rational rehabilitation plan. To locate the pathological lesion—the source of the pain—it is necessary to understand the anatomy of the nervous system, its relationship to the spine, and the biochemical process of nerve impulse transmission.

Each of the structures discussed below has characteristic pain patterns. An injury affecting spinal mechanics and structures will often cause a number of simultaneous pain patterns (e.g., facet pain and muscular pain). A detailed history of activities which affect the pain and a careful physical examination are necessary to properly diagnose the specific structures involved in an individual's injury.

THE SPINE

The spine is composed of 24 individual bones called vertebrae and a terminal bone consisting of five fused vertebrae called the sacrum (Fig. 2-1). The

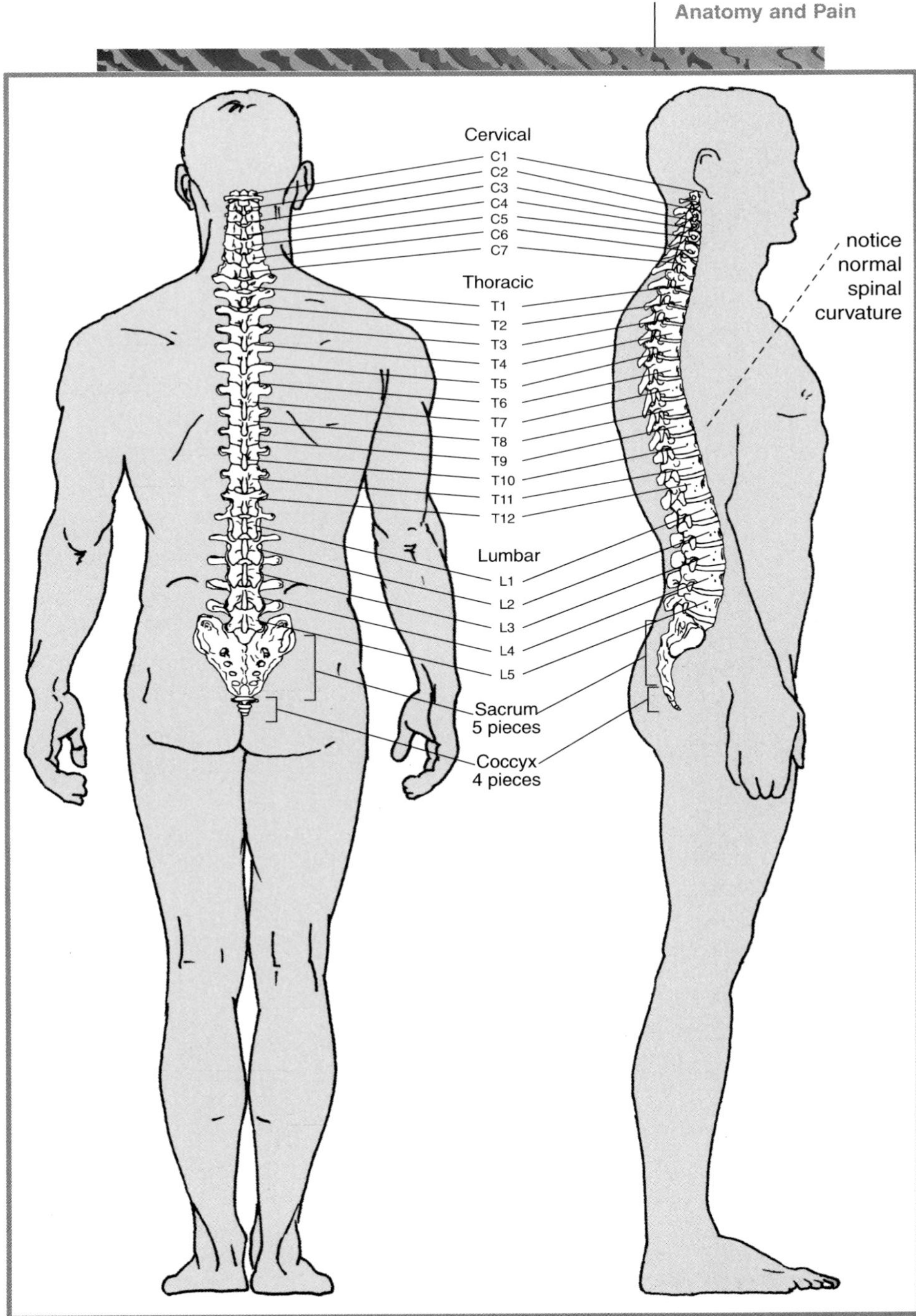

FIG. 2-1. Spine, showing 7 cervical (neck) vertebrae, 12 thoracic (chest) vertebrae, 5 lumbar (lower back) vertebrae, and sacral unit (base of spine).

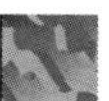

spine provides skeletal support for the entire body; without it we could not stand or even sit. In addition, the vertebrae protect the spinal cord; therefore, vertebral displacement and malalignment can have a potentially deleterious effect on the nervous system as a whole.

The spinal column consists of a series of functional units that are aligned and interlocked. Each functional unit consists of an **anteriorly** located weight-bearing component and a **posteriorly** located component which houses the spinal cord and nerve roots and determines segmental spinal motion (Fig. 2-2). The anterior component is weight-bearing and shock-absorbing, consisting of vertebral bodies segmented by an intervertebral disc. The disc prevents the vertebrae from grinding on each other. The posterior component consists of the **facets**, spinous process, transverse process, and the ligaments and muscle attachments which protect the neural structures within the spinal canal. The posterior component also limits motion via articulation of the facets.

The disc contains 88% water, and under normal circumstances can function as a shock absorber and hold the vertebrae apart. With aging and disease, water is lost from the discs, and the vertebrae can come closer together. Also, especially with rotation (twist tension or torque; Fig. 2-3), the annular fibers can be overstretched and may tear. The nucleus can then herniate, or protrude through the broken boundary of the disc fibers (Fig. 2-2C), when placed under sufficient pressure. Fluid from the nucleus is very irritating and can initiate a cascade of chemical reactions leading to inflammation of the tissue surrounding the adjacent spinal nerve. Therefore, disc material can cause inflammation of pain-sensitive structures by two mechanisms: 1) direct neural compression, and 2) chemical inflammation.

The facets form joints that act as interlocking gears between two vertebrae. These joints allow

anterior: front

posterior: back

facet: small smooth area on bone

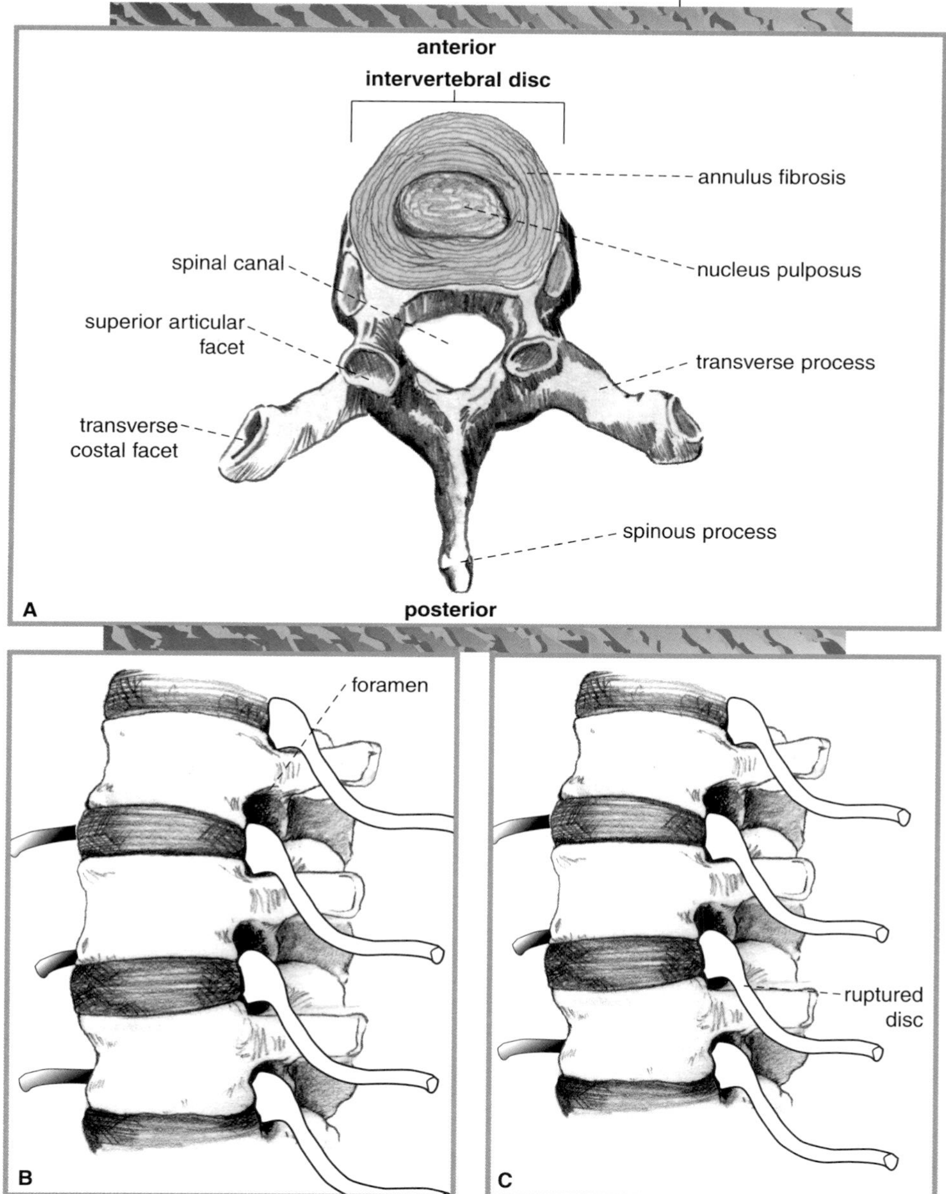

FIG. 2-2. A) Cross section of sixth thoracic vertebra and intervertebral disc, showing central nucleus with ring-shaped layer of connective tissue forming the annulus around the outside. The fibers of the annulus attach around the cartilage plates of the vertebra at a cross angle to reinforce the disc. B) Side view of spine, with nerve roots exiting between vertebrae. The annulus forms a joint above and below each vertebra. C) Herniated disc pinching on nerve root.

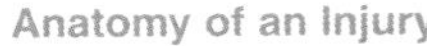

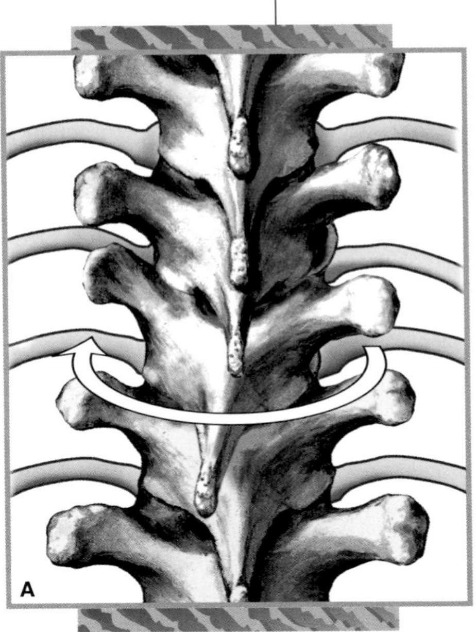

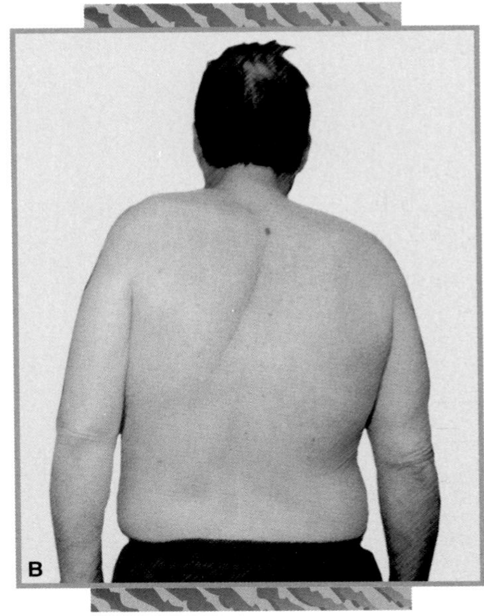

FIG. 2-3. A) Rotation of vertebra, which can result in pinched nerve. B) Patient with rotation of thoracic spine after injury.

forward and backward spinal movement in the lumbar area (**flexion** and **extension**) and forward, backward, and rotational movement in the thoracic and cervical areas. These joints also limit motion in a variety of directions to maintain stability. Facet joints of the spine, like other joints, have cartilage, capsule, joint fluid, and ligaments, and they are lubricated with synovial fluid. The joints contain pain fibers and proprioception fibers, and when injured, they can become inflamed, causing pain and altered vertebral alignment.

LIGAMENTS

Stability of vertebral alignment and coordinated movement require connections between the functional units. This connection is formed by spinal ligaments (Fig. 2-4).

flexion: bending forward

extension: bending backward

Ligaments, which are tough bands of collagen tissue with limited ability to stretch, stabilize the spine for proper weight-bearing. The ligaments contain sensory nerves that relay pain if the ligament is injured and **proprioceptive** nerve fibers which give information about spinal alignment. Torn or stretched spinal ligaments are a frequent source of pain. Chiropractic and osteopathic theory of vertebral alignment is based upon the understanding that ligaments as well as the muscles surrounding the joints have pain nerves as well as proprioceptive nerves. This concept is important to remember when we discuss treatment.

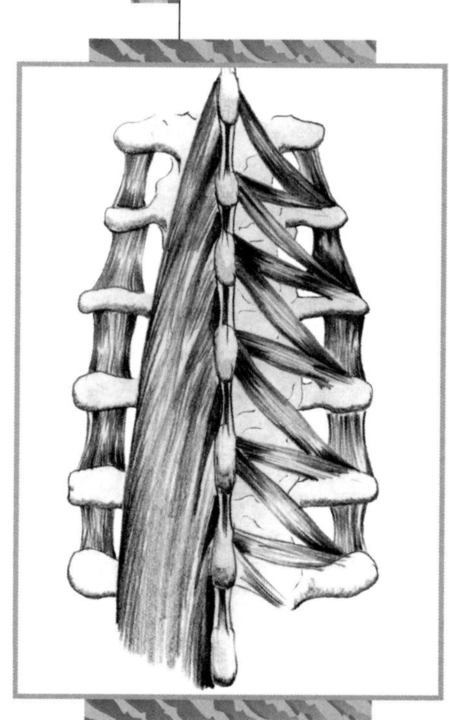

FIG. 2-4. Spine with ligaments connecting vertebrae.

THE SPINAL CANAL

The spinal canal is a tube that runs within the vertebral column from the base of the skull to the tailbone and is the conduit for the spinal cord (see Fig. 2-2A). The canal allows the passage of nerve roots to and from the spinal cord at each functional unit.

NERVE ROOTS

A nerve root (radicula) is a group of nerve fibers that carry sensory and motor impulses to and from the spinal cord, joints, muscles, and skin of the periphery (the arms, legs, and trunk). Each nerve root emerges from the spinal cord through an opening (foramen) on both sides of the spinal canal between a pair of vertebrae (Fig. 2-2B). The nerve root is covered by the **dural** sac, the protective sheath

proprioception: subconscious awareness of the body's position and movement in space

dura: the fibrous membrane enclosing the brain and spinal cord

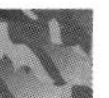

around the brain, spinal cord, and nerve roots, which contains spinal fluid and blood supply. From the nerve root emerges a small nerve branch that innervates back muscles, joints, and ligaments of the spine. Sensory information from pain-sensitive spinal structures travels back to the spinal cord via the nerve roots.

With normal anatomy and movement, the foramen widens with flexion and narrows with extension without pinching the nerve root—therefore no pain. However, if the disc herniates, taking up space in the foramen, or a bone spur grows into the foramen, the nerve root can be pinched (Fig. 2-2C), causing radicular pain.

Each sensory root of the spinal cord innervates a specific anatomical area, as shown in Figure 2-5. Thus, nerve root pain and dysfunction can be specifically identified. This is known as a **dermatomal** distribution of abnormal sensation (i.e., a pattern of specific nerve root distribution). In addition, each nerve root has a motor division which supplies specific muscles. With nerve root pathology, testing of these specific muscles might show weakness and dysfunction. This is known as a **myotomal** pattern. If the patient's history and physical examination reveal severe sensory loss (numbness) and abnormal temperature sensation or motor loss (weakness) resulting from mechanical pressure on the nerve root, surgery may be necessary. Such compression can be caused by a herniated disc, a bone spur from arthritis, or a tumor, to mention only a few examples.

dermatone: area of skin supplied by single segment of spinal nerve

myotome: group of muscles supplied by single segment of spinal nerve

autonomic: the aspect of the nervous system that regulates involuntary functions

ganglion: an aggregation of nerve cell bodies in the peripheral nervous system which relay information to the central nervous system

THE AUTONOMIC NERVOUS SYSTEM

The **autonomic** nervous system consists of chains of **ganglia** (relay stations of nerve cell bodies)

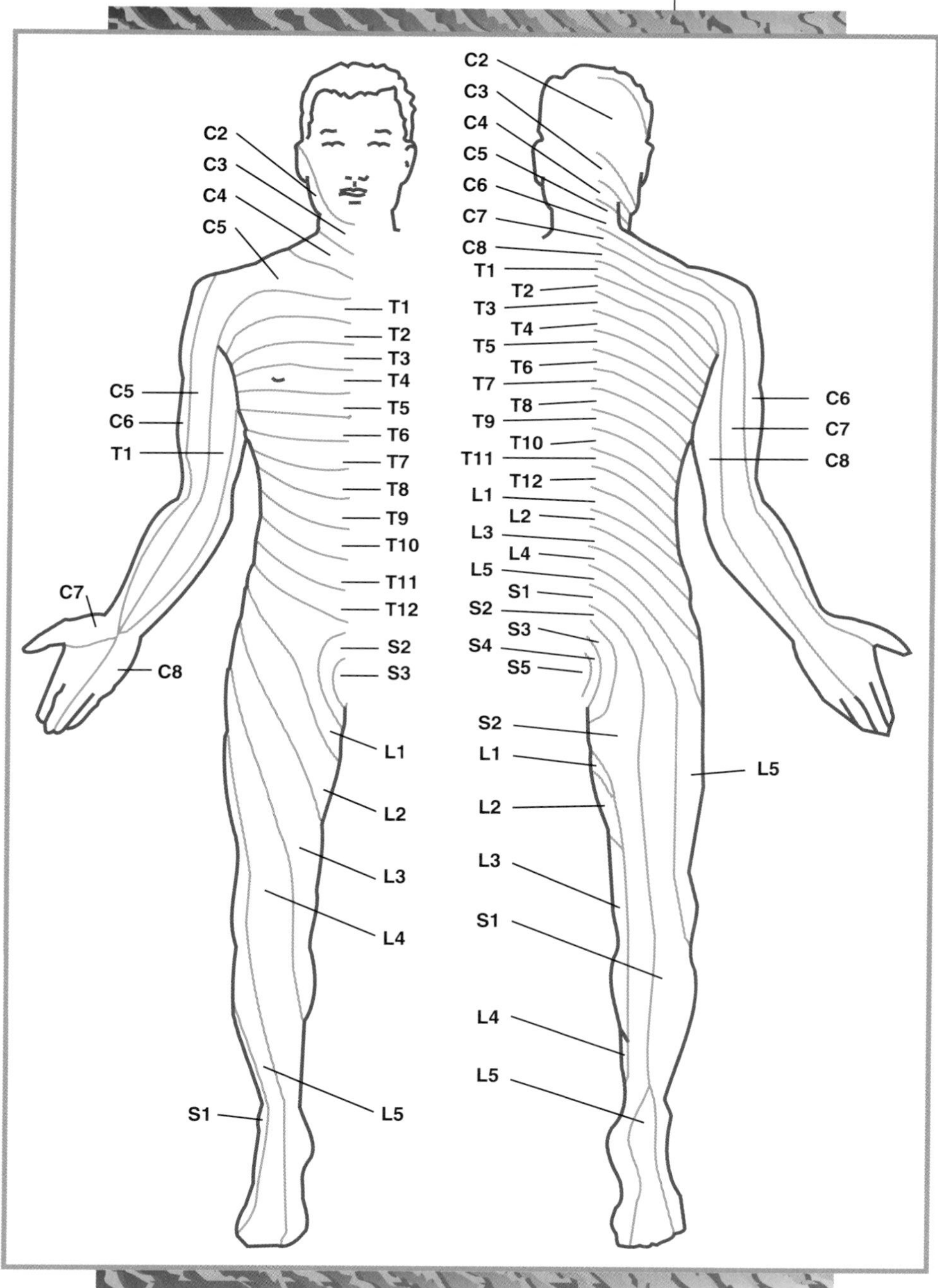

FIG. 2-5. Areas of the body supplied by each nerve root.

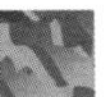

which arise from fibers from the spinal cord. It relays information through the nervous system via interlaced neural pathways. Nerve fibers from the autonomic nervous system also interface with the spinal nerve at the dorsal root ganglia (Fig. 2-6).

The autonomic nervous system controls such involuntary bodily functions as sweating, salivation, and heart rate. It can both slow down and initiate physical functions. The two parts of the autonomic nervous system are the sympathetic (thoracolumbar) and the parasympathetic (craniosacral).

Nerve fibers of the sympathetic system arise from the thoracic spinal cord and are grouped together to form twenty-three pairs of ganglia along the front of the vertebrae. Sympathetic fibers travel from the cervical ganglia to the head and face and from the thoracic and lumbar ganglia to organs of the chest and abdomen. The ganglia allow information in the sympathetic chain to be relayed to different levels of the spinal cord and from one side of the body to the other. This means that the place where sensations are felt can be different from their source.

The sympathetic nervous system helps regulate internal organ function and body energy distribution via chemical messengers. Energy distribution is regulated by the timely shunting of blood to active organs or muscles. With damage to the sympathetic nervous system, inappropriate changes in blood flow can cause low energy states to exist in muscles with resulting dysfunction, decreased elasticity, and eventually pain. Poor blood flow to fingers and toes can cause pain similar to that seen in people with atherosclerosis and frost bite. In the case of sympathetic nerve dysfunction, the blood vessels may be normal, with the problem being regulation of blood flow.

The parasympathetic system, which consists of nerve fibers from cranial nerves and from the sacral

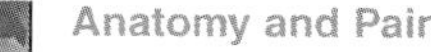

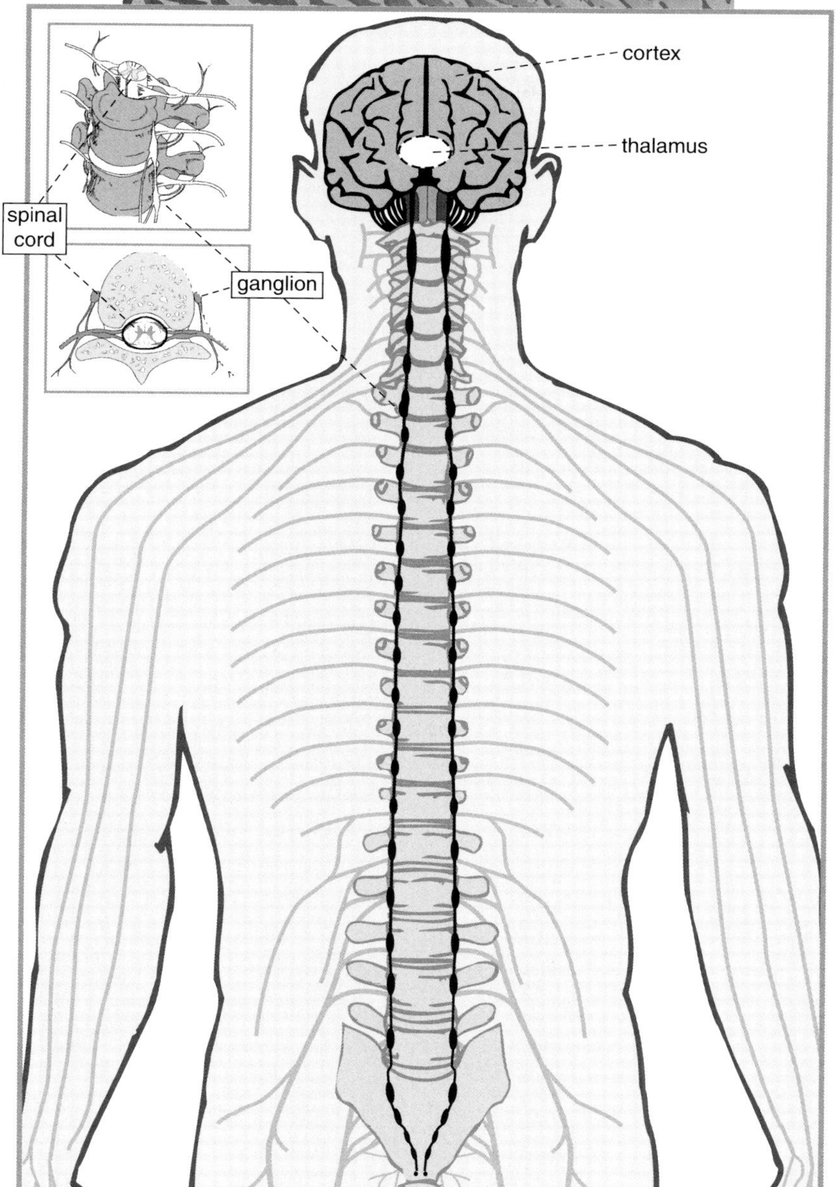

FIG. 2-6. Ganglia to sympathetic nervous system. Insets: Relationship of ganglia to vertebrae and spinal cord.

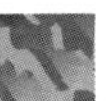

part of the spinal cord, generally produces the opposite physiological effect from the sympathetic. For example, while the sympathetic nervous system tends to accelerate heart rate, decrease salivary secretion, and increase blood pressure by constricting blood vessels, the parasympathetic system does the reverse. Thus the two parts of the autonomic system function in a complementary way.

When pain sensations are transmitted to the brain, two sites of perception receive the information. One site, in the **cortex**, localizes and characterizes the pain (e.g., sharp pain in the hand). The other site, the **thalamus**, assigns an emotional sensation to the pain (e.g., fear, anger, depression). This information is processed and refined throughout the brain and spinal cord until a final response is formulated. Recent research indicates that in chronic pain a variety of central nervous system locations can become sensitized to the constant flow of negative impulses throughout the nervous system. This causes seemingly exaggerated physical and emotional responses to minor painful stimuli. Nerve fibers from both the sympathetic and parasympathetic systems are interconnected anatomically and functionally with the peripheral and the central nervous systems. Such complicated neural relationships make understanding pain pathways very difficult.

In an injury caused by a fall, there may be initial inflammation with swelling, redness, and pain at the site of the injury. The damaged tissues release chemical mediators which continue the inflammatory response. In the injured area, nociceptors—nerves that sense and transmit painful stimuli—relay information through afferent fibers (nerves that transmit impulses from the peripheral toward the central nervous system) to the dorsal root ganglia of the spinal nerve (see Fig. 1-3). The dorsal root ganglia

cerebral cortex: outer layer of brain, governing motor, sensory, and auditory functions

thalamus: mass of brain cells that relays sensory messages to the cortex

are relay stations made up of a collection of sensory cell bodies from the spinal nerve and cell bodies from the sympathetic aspect of the autonomic nervous system. The information then enters the dorsal horn of the spinal cord through the spinal nerve at the level where the nerve segment enters the spinal cord. Through complicated pathways in the spinal cord and brain, the information is processed to either inhibit or enhance the response to pain.

CONCLUSION

Although pain can have various causes (such as muscle spasm or a crushed nerve), most of the pain we treat originates with tension on the nervous system. For example, vertebrae out of normal alignment cause pain in several ways. One mechanism, of course, is pressure on a nerve root, or radicular pain. When a nerve root is aggravated, a typical dermatomal pattern of pain referral (see Fig. 2-5) is seen, and muscles supplied by the nerve root can become dysfunctional. But pain may also arise from tension placed on vertebrae, facet joints, and spinal ligaments. When these structures become inflamed and/or placed under tension, a typical well-described pain pattern referred from each vertebral segment can be noted. When a vertebral rotation is left untreated, a secondary counterrotation at another level can develop in response to regular use and/or minor trauma. This can lead to pain at a distant site, as well as muscular dysfunction, which in turn leads to pain that "spreads" and/or is disproportionate to the original injury.

There are some cases of chronic pain with no obvious source of injury. Just as physicians can diagnose neurological diseases such as multiple sclerosis but cannot yet offer patients a cure, so must we bear in mind that although many sources

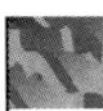

of pain can be identified, there remain obscure and complicated pain syndromes we cannot describe, anatomically or functionally. As neural pathways and relays become more clearly defined, physicians will be better able to identify causes of pain and thus develop more effective treatment.

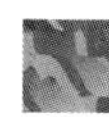

3 Myofascial Pain

Myofascial pain is a common, treatable soft-tissue disorder. Other terms used to describe myofascial pain are fibromyositis, muscular rheumatism, fibromyalgia, and myogelosis.

Myofascial pain is the most misunderstood and mismanaged of all pain and injury problems. Although there are over 400 muscles in the human body, composing 40% of the body weight, the study of muscle dysfunction is skimmed over quickly in medical school curricula. Today, however, extensive information on myofascial pain is being documented through research—and evidence shows that it can be highly responsive to treatment.

Myofascial pain is highly responsive to treatment.

In pure myofascial pain syndromes, diagnostic tests such as MRI or CT scan of the spine may show nothing abnormal. There is, however, a diagnostic hallmark for myofascial pain—the trigger point. Normal muscles do not contain trigger points. Observations of patients and experimental evidence all suggest that a myofascial trigger point begins with muscular overload. It may start abruptly after a car accident or insidiously as a patient decreases range of motion through aging and lifestyle changes.

myofascial: relating to muscles and connective tissue

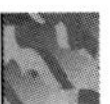

TRIGGER POINTS

A trigger point, which is a contracted band of muscle fibers, is a site of localized ischemia (decreased blood flow) which causes irritability of nerve endings. When activated, the trigger point transmits pain to a distant zone (Fig. 3-1). The trigger point and not the distant zone is the source of pain. This referred pain is characteristic for the particular trigger point and can occur while the muscle is either at rest or in motion. An active trigger point is always tender, prevents full lengthening of the muscle, and may cause weakness or easy fatigability in addition to pain. Certain trigger points can activate the sympathetic nervous system and produce other phenomena in the referred pain zone, such as vasoconstriction (blanching), coldness, sweating, and eyelid droop. The severity of referred symptoms ranges from painless restriction of motion caused by inactive trigger points to agonizing, incapacitating pain.

Trigger points are located at the motor end plate of the muscle (i.e., where the nerves supplying these muscles enter the muscle). These locations are the same in all people and are well described in trigger point maps and manuals published by Travell and Simons. When examining a patient for trigger points, the physician searches these locations to identify a small palpable band of muscle approximately 1/8" in size. This tender band, when stimulated, by either strumming the fibers and/or causing a contraction in a specific muscle, will yield the typical referred pain pattern.

Active trigger points are most likely to occur in postural muscles of the neck, shoulder, and pelvis. The more hypersensitive the trigger point, the more intense and constant the referred pain and the more extensive the distribution of the pain. Trigger points

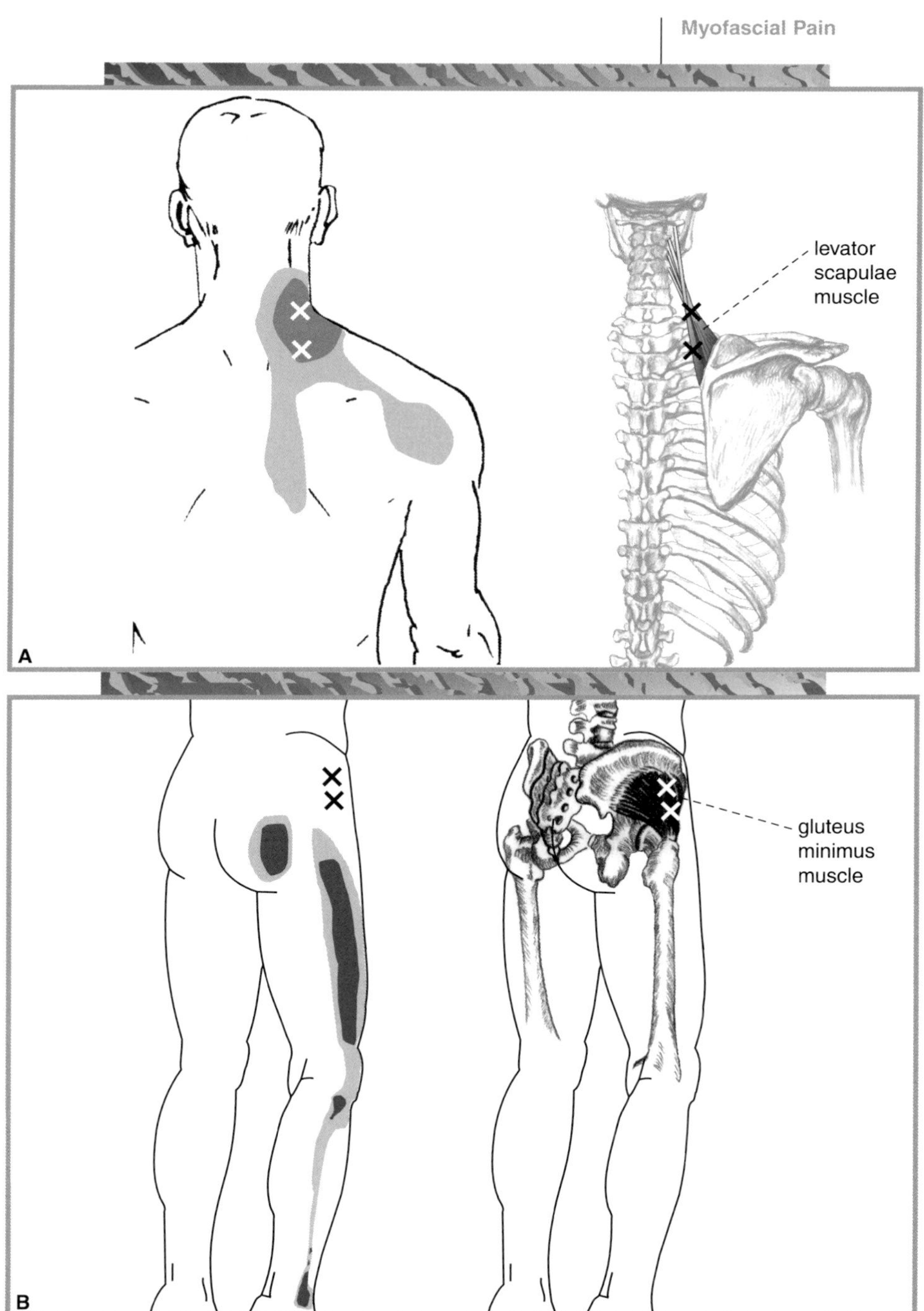

FIG. 3-1. Patterns of referred pain. A) Trigger points in the neck (levator scapulae muscle). B) Trigger points in the hip (gluteus minimus muscle).

are activated in two ways: 1) directly, by overwork, fatigue, direct trauma, and chilling; and 2) indirectly, by other trigger points and underlying diseases such as appendicitis, arthritis, and emotional distress. Weakness from trigger points may be caused when messages from the central nervous system are inhibited as a way of protecting the muscle from achieving a painful degree of contraction. The patient then substitutes other muscles to compensate for the weak one, and eventually, as described in Chapter 1, the compensation causes abnormal movement patterns. Figure 3-1 shows how a trigger point in one area of the body refers pain to a distant area. Just as pulling the trigger of a gun affects a remote target, so activation of a trigger point projects pain at a distance. Such patterns of pain invariably can be reproduced by applying pressure to the trigger point and so are completely predictable.

Certainly, not all pain syndromes are purely myofascial in origin. People do have herniated discs, fractured bones, and undetected brain tumors. However, most pain syndromes have an associated myofascial component since pain causes muscle dysfunction. Very often, it is this component, left untreated, that can be most frustrating to the patient. For example, a physician may mistakenly focus on the site of the pain rather than on its remote source, for example, overlooking the muscles in the back, which insert on the shoulder and cause pain experienced in the shoulder. Or the physician may operate on the back and remove a herniated disc or repair a fractured bone, assuming the pain will automatically disappear. When pain continues because the myofascial component has been ignored, the physician may tell the patient that he or she "just has to live with it."

Activities such as stretching and conditioning actually decrease pain.

The body's primitive response to pain is withdrawal, and when injury occurs, muscles contract. If injury is severe, the contraction is sustained and trigger points develop. Left untreated, these abnormally contracted muscles perpetuate a pain cycle.

When patients mistakenly believe they have to "just live with it," they may feel hopeless and restrict their activity to avoid pain. Patient education is essential to alleviate the fear that movement poses a risk of further damage. Activities such as stretching and conditioning actually decrease myofascial pain by releasing contracted muscle. Patient education must also emphasize that myofascial pain is treatable. For example, if someone having chest pain thinks they are having a heart attack, they may feel terrified and helpless. But if they are taught that in reality their chest pain is from a chest muscle trigger point, this knowledge will alleviate their fear, decrease the pain, and enable them to take a proactive role in their recovery. The perception of pain is intimately related to the patient's understanding of the underlying source. Thus, education is indispensable.

OTHER SOURCES OF MUSCULOSKELETAL PAIN

There are three major categories of musculoskeletal diseases that must be distinguished from pure myofascial trigger point pain. These are myopathies, arthritis, and inflammations such as tendinitis and bursitis.

Myopathies

Myopathies are usually marked by painless weakness of proximal girdle muscles (those close to the trunk). If pain is present, it is usually minor,

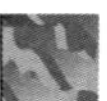

whereas with myofascial trigger points, pain is the chief complaint. Examples of myopathies are polymyositis and dermatomyositis. Polymyositis usually begins as a painless weakness of certain limb muscles, with little evidence of systemic infection, and can progress to total paralysis. Dermatomyositis resembles polymyositis but has associated skin changes, including erythema (redness), maculopapular eruption (rash), and eczema. A lilac color over the bridge of the nose, cheeks, and forehead and around fingernails helps identify dermatomyositis. Muscle enzyme levels which are within normal limits in myofascial trigger point pain syndromes are increased in both forms of myositis. Other common myopathies are polymyalgia rheumatica and temporal arteritis.

Arthritis

Pain referred from myofascial trigger points can closely mimic the pain of osteoarthritis, rheumatoid arthritis, psoriatic arthritis, and gout. Myofascial pain referred to a joint is often misdiagnosed as arthritis. In general, arthritis can be diagnosed from local signs such as crepitation (crackling sound), restriction of movement, and instability in the joint. Osteoarthritis, or degenerative joint disease, involves degeneration of cartilage in a joint. Its diagnosis rests primarily on local joint pain, tenderness with crepitation, degeneration of cartilage, and bone degeneration documented by x-ray examination. Bone spurs, lipping (the formation of a overlapping edge of bone in a joint), and joint space narrowing noted on x-ray film (Fig. 3-2) are *not* specific to the diagnosis of osteoarthritis. Most patients who have arthritis also have myofascial pain resulting from abnormal movement patterns associated with the arthritis. If the myofascial component is treated, these arthritic patients can experience decreased pain.

Many myofascial pain sufferers are told erroneously that their pain is caused by arthritis and that there may be no effective treatment. However, it is myofascial pain, not arthritis, when there are trigger points and a smoothly moving joint. It is important to know that most of these patients become pain-free when trigger points are deactivated.

Many myofascial pain sufferers are told that their pain is caused by arthritis, but most of them become pain-free when trigger points are deactivated.

Rheumatoid arthritis is a **systemic** disease. The hallmark of rheumatoid arthritis is proliferation of synovium (joint membrane) which spreads over the joint surface and damages cartilage, bone, and joint capsule. The American Rheumatological Association recommends that the diagnosis be made if seven of these eleven criteria are met: morning stiffness, joint pain, joint swelling, symmetrical joint swelling, nodules under the skin, x-ray changes, fatigue, low-grade fever, positive blood test for rheumatoid factor, protein precipitates in synovial fluid, and joint tissue changes noted on slides. Women are affected three times more often than men. The diagnosis of gouty arthritis is made by finding urate crystals in synovial fluid samples. Psoriatic arthritis is an inflammatory arthritis (swollen joints) with the skin and nail lesions of psoriasis. Patients suffering from pure myofascial pain syndromes will have none of these positive diagnostic findings.

Tendinitis and Bursitis

Because myofascial pain is referred to regions where **tendons** and **bursae** are located, it is frequently misdiagnosed as tendinitis or bursitis, or inflammation of those areas. In true bursitis, the skin over the joint appears as hot, red, and swollen. At the time the bursa is evaluated, the muscles should be examined for active trigger points. Joint inflammation, bursitis, and/or tendonitis need to be differentiated from myofascial

systemic: affecting the whole body rather than a single part

tendon: fibrous band of tissue that attaches muscle to bone

bursa: fibrous cushion that allows tendon to move smoothly over bone

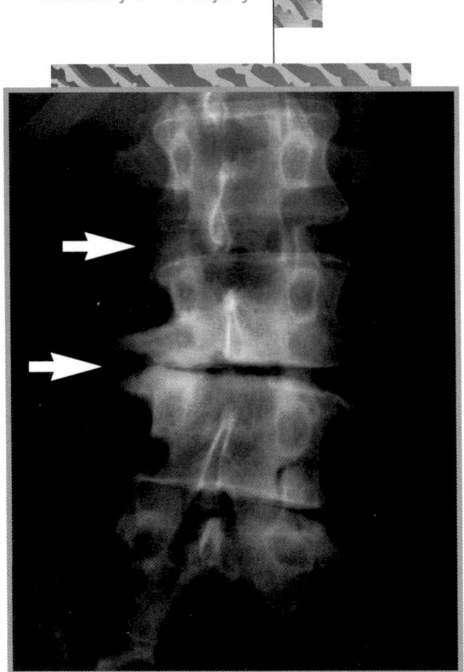

FIG. 3-2. X-ray film showing normal joint (top arrow) and arthritic joint (bottom arrow) in lumbar spine. Notice loss of alignment in arthritic joint.

pain syndromes and treated with localized injection and anti-inflammatory medication, often steroids.

DIAGNOSIS AND TREATMENT

The diagnosis of myofascial pain is made by careful and complete examination. The muscle, instead of being smooth, symmetrical, and supple has palpable taut bands that, when pressed, may cause a twitch or a pattern of pain referred to a distant area. Usually myofascial pain is aggravated by cold, viral infection, and direct trauma. Patients feel worse in the morning because of decreased movement during sleep. Myofascial pain is lessened by rest, aggressive stretching, and moist heat.

The key to treatment of myofascial pain is to deactivate the trigger point.Various approaches are effective. If the pain is moderately severe and of short duration, the pain syndrome may respond to manual physical therapy or myofascial release physical therapy. Spray-and-stretch, a technique in which the patient is passively stretched after a vapocoolant anesthetic is sprayed over the muscle, also can be effective. Ischemic compression, which has long been advocated by massage therapists, involves firmly pressing the trigger point with the fingers until the muscle is felt to release and the band disappears. Treatment with ultrasound also may deactivate trigger points, but we have not found it nearly as effective as aggressive manual therapy which corrects underlying structural abnormalities by releasing tightness in muscles that pull the body out of proper alignment.

By far the most effective treatment in the deactivation of trigger points is injection (in the trigger point) of 1-2 cc. of 0.5% Xylocaine (a local anesthetic) to relax contracted muscle fibers. Xylocaine also dilates blood vessels, thus increasing blood flow to the muscle. Hot packs applied to a muscle directly after trigger point injection decrease postinjection soreness as heat increases blood flow and relaxation. Relief is more likely to be lasting when the treated muscles are stretched through their full range of motion to eliminate trigger points. This also helps the patient relearn normal movement and have less tendency to guard against pain. The injections have been microscopically shown to cause a breakdown of the abnormal muscle fibers, which allows for regeneration of new tissue. This process takes about seven days to occur, and therefore injection of the trigger point should not be performed more than once a week.

Aggressive manual therapy can correct underlying structural abnormalities by releasing tightness in muscles that pull the body out of proper alignment.

Because underlying structural abnormalities affect body function, it is important to understand what muscle actions and what movements and stress situations are likely to activate and perpetuate trigger points. Sustained postural overload and poor work habits need to be corrected. So do impaired circulation and dietary inadequacies; folic acid is essential to energy and metabolism, and anemia, hypoglycemia, and inadequate thyroid hormone can aggravate the myofascial pain syndrome. Of course, underlying infectious diseases, neurological diseases, major organ dysfunctions, and neoplasms must be treated. More frequently, a patient's lifestyle, anxieties, coping behavior, and understanding of symptoms all affect the pain. Each of these contributing aspects should be treated individually but simultaneously.

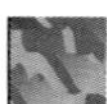

Some centers advocate injection of steroid into the trigger point, either in conjunction with local anesthetic or alone. There is evidence that this is more effective than local anesthetic alone but carries the downside of steroid side effects such as weight gain, adrenal suppression, and hyperglycemia. Furthermore, steroids injected in the superficial layers of the skin can cause depigmentation of the skin. There are also those who prefer to simply "dry needle" the trigger point—that is, to place the needle into the trigger point without injecting anything. We feel this is less effective and also causes greater postinjection soreness. Therefore, we inject trigger points with local anesthetic and find the temporary numbness facilitates physical therapy.

There are few complications of trigger point injections; these include postinjection soreness, localized infection, allergic reactions, inadvertent puncture of the lung, and intravascular injection. Use of sterile technique and preservative-free anesthetics greatly limits infection and allergic reactions. The small dose involved limits the risk of intravascular injection. The greatest risk is of inadvertent puncture—particularly of the lung when injecting trigger points of the chest, upper back, and the base of the neck—but this can be minimized by using a short, small-gauge needle.

PART II
DIAGNOSIS

"God whispers to us in our pleasures, speaks in our conscience, but shouts in our pain..."

C. S. Lewis,
The Problem of Pain

4 THE INITIAL EXAMINATION

Taking a patient's medical history and conducting a physical examination initiates a relationship between patient and physician. Often patients are wary because previous physicians found no medical reason and offered no treatment for their pain. Thus, during the interview, it is important that trust be established. The rehabilitative process will be a new and at times painful experience, requiring the patient's full participation and compliance with the home exercise program. The physician also should bear in mind that trust must be earned, making patience, education, and communication essential tools.

Because chronic pain is often related to a previous injury or underlying disease, it is important that patients include minor accidents and illnesses as part of their history.

HISTORY

The medical history consists of all the relevant information the patient can give the physician about the problem that brought him or her to seek treatment. Because chronic pain is often related to a previous injury or underlying disease process, it is important that patients not overlook past experiences, such as minor accidents or disease, as part of their history. Likewise, information about hobbies, such as sports

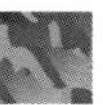

activities, playing a musical instrument, or spending hours at a computer, can contribute to understanding trauma from repetitive movement. The physician must explain how cause and effect can operate over long periods of time so the patient can understand how an old injury may lead to current pain. As we like to say, "We are the sum of our traumas."

A history of previous surgical procedures is also important. A patient may be experiencing pain from internal as well as external scars. Scars can trap nerves, causing severe pain. Patients also may have pain caused by having been in an awkward position on the operating table. For example, persistent chest wall pain in people who have had spinal fusion may have begun when they were placed face down on a large metal frame for an extended time period during surgery—a cause that is often overlooked. Although the patient was asleep, the body was experiencing major physiological stress that had a lasting effect.

Soft-tissue pain varies in intensity and location, depending on the activity of trigger points.

It is important to describe pain as specifically as possible—dull, aching, burning, stabbing, tingling, or cramping—because the quality of the pain often is the first diagnostic clue. The patient may be reluctant to say that the pain is not always consistent in location or intensity for fear the physician will not find him or her credible. Nerve root (discogenic) pain occurs in a consistent pattern because it follows a dermatome or particular area of skin supplied by a single spinal nerve (see Fig. 2-5). Soft-tissue pain, on the other hand, varies in intensity and location, depending on the activity of trigger points.

The physician must consider drug allergies and carefully review often complicated medical regimens. Pain medications, particularly narcotics, must be cautiously dispensed to avoid dependence. The health

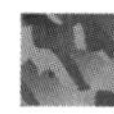

care team and the patient share a responsibility to ensure that there is no duplication of prescriptions from another physician. However, patients with cancer or severe untreatable pain syndromes should be offered relief from their pain—if necessary, with daily narcotics. In situations in which rehabilitation may not decrease pain, appropriate narcotic medications can enhance the quality of life.

Questions about various aspects of the patient's life, such as changes in daily habits, recreation, and family activities, may reveal relevant information. For example, if sleep patterns are disturbed by pain, early normalization of sleep may be essential to full recovery. We ask about losses in recreational activity to evaluate not only the extent of the injury but also to assess personal goals. Often family relationships deteriorate if parents cannot play with young children or enjoy family vacations because of pain. It is important to at least start to understand family dynamics during evaluation, so the physician can identify and enlist the aid of supportive family members or structure a treatment plan independent of frustrated or angry family members.

The sensation of pain is a learned experience. Patients' previous painful diseases or injuries can affect their current pain problem by causing them to either exaggerate or down-play the reports of pain intensity. For example, a patient who has recently been treated for cancer pain may associate new aches and dysfunctions with the cancer, thereby escalating his or her complaints.

Thoroughness is essential in the history-taking process. Illness may cause or exacerbate pain syndromes. Patient education must address potential limitations in the rehabilitative process caused by coexisting conditions. For example:

- Diabetics (particularly poorly controlled

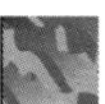

diabetics) are prone to develop thick, coarse, edematous skin, and this connective tissue distortion may limit range of motion.

- Cancer symptoms may develop insidiously; people with swollen ankles may be suffering from a tumor in the pelvis.
- Hormonal disorders, particularly hypothyroidism, are associated with increased incidence of myofascial pain.
- Patients with collagen vascular diseases, such as lupus or rheumatoid arthritis, may benefit from manual therapy techniques, but chronic use of steroids for these conditions may cause thin skin and fragile bones.

A complete evaluation of the patient enables the physician to design a treatment program within the patient's capacity to adapt.

PHYSICAL EXAMINATION

The physical examination includes a neurological evaluation to distinguish between spinal cord damage and soft-tissue injury.

The physical examination includes a neurological evaluation to distinguish between nerve root or spinal cord damage and soft-tissue or peripheral injury. For example, if a person cannot stand on their toes or drags a foot while walking, this may indicate compression of a lumbar nerve root. One calf muscle that is much thinner than the other may be caused by a movement disorder or by nerve root damage. Reflex changes in the upper and lower extremities reveal patterns of nerve dysfunction that enable the physician to isolate nerve roots at specific levels of the spinal cord as the source of pain.

The patient's structural alignment also is examined in detail. Since the pelvis is a major supportive structure of the body, it is important that it be level

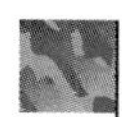

and centered. Body alignment from head to feet is analyzed for symmetry and movement. Severely pronated (flat) feet can easily be treated with an inexpensive arch support, and such a simple intervention may reduce back and neck pain. **Palpation** is used to evaluate muscles and skin for elasticity and firmness and to identify specific trigger points.

The vertebrae are carefully analyzed for rotation or displacement that creates a deviation from normal spinal curvatures. Since the nerve roots exit between the vertebrae, spinal malalignment is a major cause of mechanical pain. Specific maneuvers of muscle groups help identify improperly aligned vertebrae. Analysis of alignment in standing, sitting, and lying down reveals postural defects and muscle imbalances. Identification of these imbalances can yield information concerning the pattern of injury.

Movement analysis evaluates the functioning of major muscle groups. Patients suffering from back pain commonly have gluteal (buttocks) muscles that are flaccid (lacking firmness and resilience). In such cases, muscle testing maneuvers may reveal premature irregular contraction of low back muscles to compensate for nonfunctioning gluteal muscles. This aggravates back pain. Not only strengthening gluteal muscles but also training them to work in the correct sequence is essential to relieve the pain.

Physical examination of surgical scars identifies fascial **constriction**. Manual release of constriction through various layers of scar tissue will result in increased range of motion. Previous surgery is important also because disruption of normal anatomy may prevent complete recovery from pain. In such cases, it is important to set realistic goals.

Not only does the physical examination give the physician the opportunity to categorize an injury, it also gives patients an opportunity to learn how

palpation: examination by sensitive placement of the physician's hands on the patient's body

constriction: abnormal binding or tightness of the connective tissue

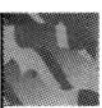

structural abnormalities affect their pain. Often the physical examination process may be a very positive experience for the patient as the physician documents structural and functional abnormalities that are treatable.

CONCLUSION

The initial examination is only the beginning of an ongoing conversation not only among patient, physician, and therapists but within the patient's body as well. As therapy begins, structural adjustments cause new symptoms. Movement patterns will change, determining subsequent phases of therapy. Some patients will progress quickly along a well-traveled path. Others, more pained and more wounded, will need ongoing nurturing and support. But with knowledge and will, all patients can move from this starting point towards wellness.

5 Testing

Although there is much art in medicine, the decision to order a test should be based on science and logic. When a test is ordered, the physician is responsible for knowing the cost of the test and what information the test is intended to reveal. Technological improvements offer more and more information, but not all information is relevant to a given patient's problem. Also, test results are not always accurate or clinically significant. The physician needs to order a test based on his/her evaluation of the patient and render treatment based on the results of the test.

Technological improvements offer more and more information, but not all information is relevant to a given patient's problem. A test should be ordered only when it is needed to gather information not otherwise obtainable or because the test results will affect treatment and outcome.

A test should be ordered only when it is needed to gather information not otherwise obtainable or because the test results will affect treatment and outcome. For instance, if the history and physical examination alone indicate the possibility of a herniated disc, and the patient has no neurological changes requiring urgent surgery, the first round of treatment may be nonsurgical (i.e., physical therapy and epidural steroid injections). The physician would not need to order an MRI to confirm the diagnosis. But if the initial treatment is unsuccessful, diagnostic testing may be necessary to clearly

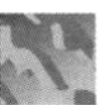

identify the problem. With the specific information provided by test results, the most appropriate mode of treatment can be determined.

There are many ways of classifying tests. The categories we use are tests of structure and tests of function. Structural tests include plain x-ray, computed tomography (CT scan), MRI scan, myelography, and bone scan. Functional tests such as nerve conduction and electromyography (EMG) evaluate nerve and muscle performance, and thermography evaluates energy or blood flow distribution. Often more than one test is necessary since each test reveals different information. The following paragraphs describe these tests.

STRUCTURAL TESTS

X-RAYS

X-rays reveal the position and integrity of bones. They can show fractures, the distance between vertebrae, loss of calcium (as from osteoporosis), or

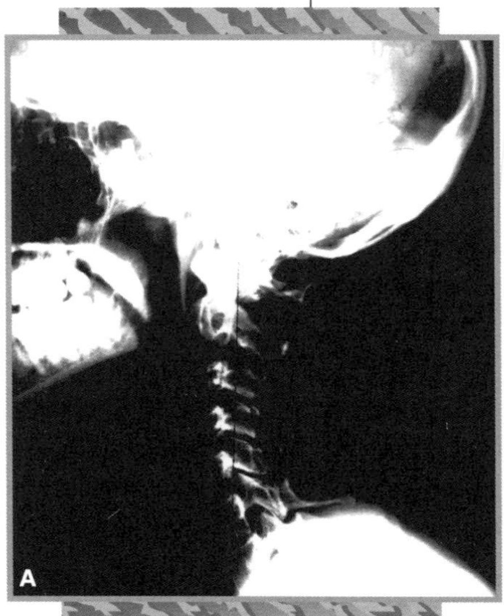

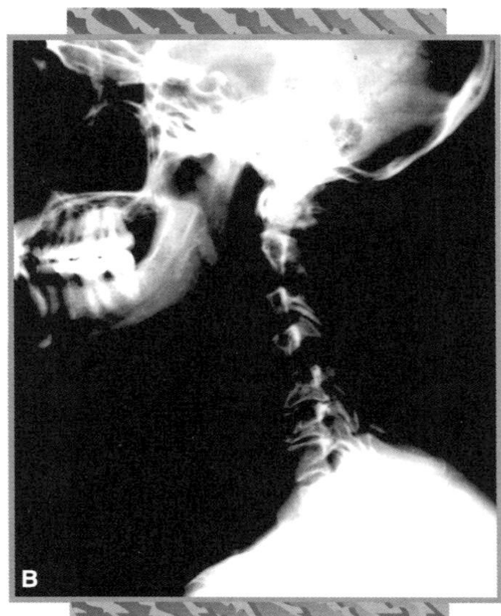

FIG. 5-1. X-ray films showing A) normal and B) abnormal cervical curves.

certain bony changes consistent with cancer. X-rays can be tests of function as well as tests of structure by taking them with the patient in different positions. For example, x-rays taken with the spine in a neutral position may show normal vertebral alignment, while those taken with the neck flexed, extended, or rotated may show an abnormal cervical curve (Fig. 5-1). By evaluating skeletal alignment during changes in position, the physician obtains an impression of joint function, or **biomechanics**. Additionally, x-rays can locate exactly the vertebral source of faulty biomechanics.

By evaluating skeletal alignment during changes in position, the physician obtains an impression of joint function.

CT Scan

Computed tomography (CT) scans provide anatomical information from cross-sectional planes of the body (Fig. 5-2). Compared to x-ray, CT gives more information about soft tissue as well as bones.

CT scans are valuable in evaluating spinal trauma. Fractures and other abnormalities of vertebral bodies and laminae can be accurately shown. Among our patients, lumbar intervertebral disc disease and spinal stenosis are frequent indications for CT scanning. CT also can demonstrate far lateral disc herniation with nerve root compression, which might be missed using

biomechanics: the study of forces exerted by muscles and gravity on a living body, or the mechanical function of a living body

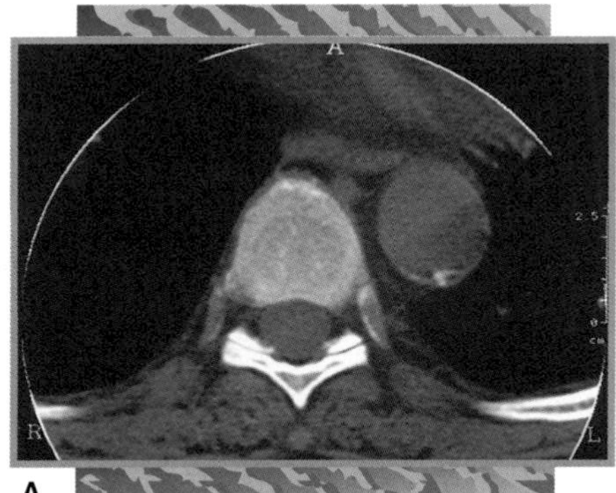

A

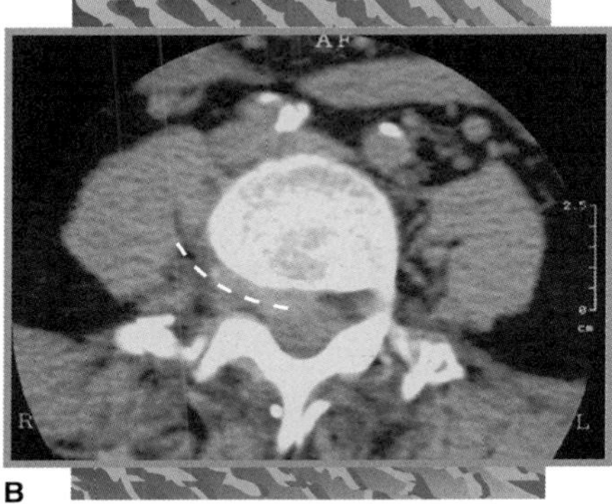

B

Figure 5-2. CT scans of cross section of vertebrae showing A) spinal canal of normal diameter, and B) herniated disc impinging on spinal canal (dashed line).

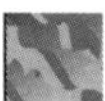

other methods. However, abnormal texture of the spinal cord cannot be detected with CT, and it is difficult to distinguish postoperative scars from recurrent disc herniation or other soft-tissue masses.

A CT scan may take 35-45 minutes.

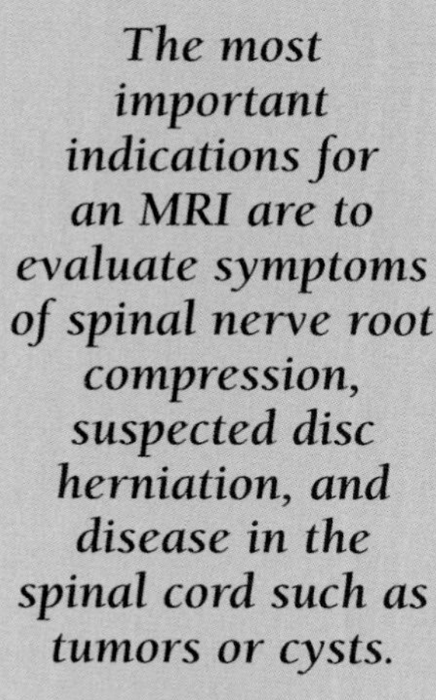

MRI Scan

Magnetic resonance imaging (MRI) is a diagnostic test utilizing magnetic properties of protons to create internal images of physical conditions not visible on x-ray film. Patients are not exposed to any form of radiation; in fact, no biological hazards from an MRI have been recorded, other than the potential of magnetic displacement of metallic implants (e.g., surgical clips placed on a cerebral aneurysm). In most instances, the MRI is better than CT for soft-tissue evaluation, and it is the most powerful, versatile technique for imaging the brain.

MRI is also an important diagnostic test for assessing the spine and spinal cord. Images can be viewed in any plane, such as coronal (dividing the body into front and back) or sagittal (dividing the body into left and right sides). Injection of intraspinal contrast medium (as in myelography, discussed below) is not necessary. Because of excellent soft-tissue resolution, it is possible to distinguish the texture of abnormal from normal spinal cord segments. Currently, the most important indications for an MRI are to evaluate symptoms of spinal nerve root compression, suspected disc herniation, and disease in the spinal cord such as tumors or cysts (Fig. 5-3).

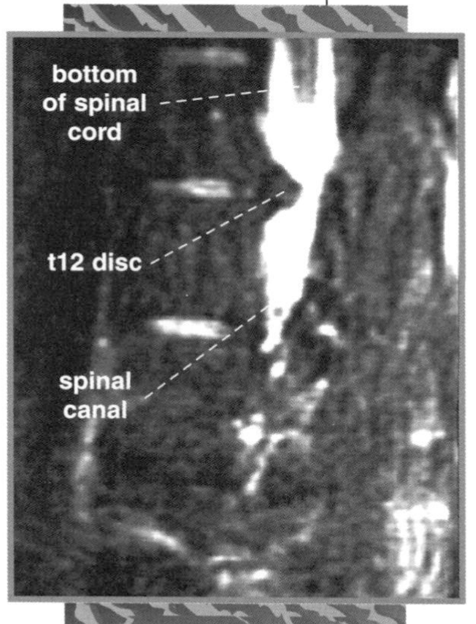

FIG. 5-3. MRI scan showing herniated disc pressing on spinal canal.

MRI does have important limitations. For example, calcification in the brain and fresh brain blood clots are poorly seen. Other drawbacks are that bone tissue produces almost no signal, making it difficult to see fractures and bone spurs. In acute trauma of the spine, CT scan is superior. Also, because metal distorts magnetic resonance, a myelogram followed by a postmyelogram CT scan are the tests of choice for evaluating the spine in patients who have large metallic implants following spinal fusion. MRI is time-consuming and requires the patient to be immobile for 45 minutes to an hour.

Myelography

A myelogram is a spinal test which evaluates the spinal cord and nerve roots. A spinal puncture is performed, followed by injection of radiopaque contrast medium around the spinal cord. This makes the spinal cord and nerve bundles look like negative shadows, as on an x-ray. Currently, water-soluble dye is used for the injection, making it easy for the dye to penetrate small crevices. Also, with water-soluble dye, removal of the contrast medium is no longer required, and complications previously associated with the dye are now less frequent.

Myelography accurately demonstrates any abnormality that causes encroachment on the spinal cord, including herniated disc, spinal stenosis, abscess, blood clot, metastatic cancer, and spinal cord tumor.

Myelography accurately demonstrates any abnormality that causes encroachment on the spinal cord, including herniated disc, spinal stenosis, abscess, blood clot, metastatic cancer, and spinal cord tumor (Fig. 5-4). However, while the presence of a lesion will be demonstrated, the extent and texture of the lesion cannot be shown by myelography.

Myelography is invasive and may be complicated by severe spinal headache, which may last a week or

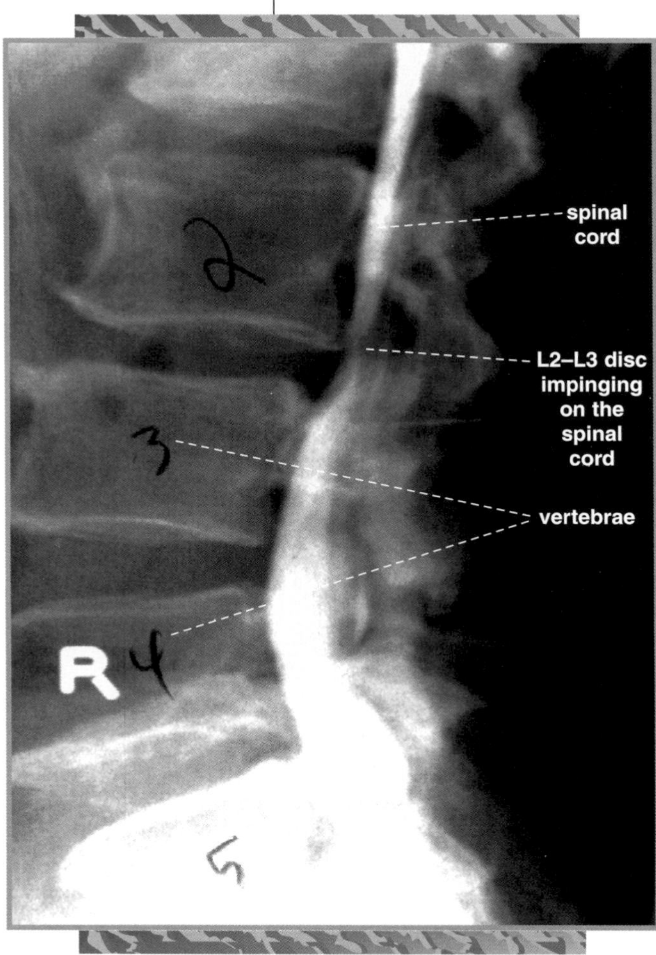

FIG. 5-4. Myelogram showing impingement of disc on spinal cord.

ten days. Myelography should not be performed on patients with seizure disorders (seizures occur in less than 1% of cases) or dye allergies (also rare). With the advent of refined techniques in CT scanning and MRI, routine myelography is discouraged. Its use is largely limited to patients scheduled for surgery to precisely locate a lesion.

Bone Scan

Bone scans detect abnormalities of bone and are frequently ordered to evaluate fractures which may not be seen on plain x-rays (Fig. 5-5). The bone scan gives information about the metabolism of the bone. It is used in diagnosis and treatment of pain problems such as osteomyelitis (bone infections), tumors which may not be revealed on plain x-rays, or reflex sympathetic dystrophy (a malfunction of the autonomic nervous system which may occur with electrical injuries, as a side effect of a major illness, or, most often, after blunt trauma to an arm or leg).

dye excreted through the urinary system appears in the bladder
dark areas of increased uptake of arthritic bone
ANTERIOR
ANTERIOR
POSTERIOR
POSTERIOI

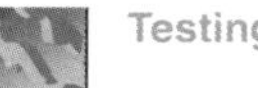

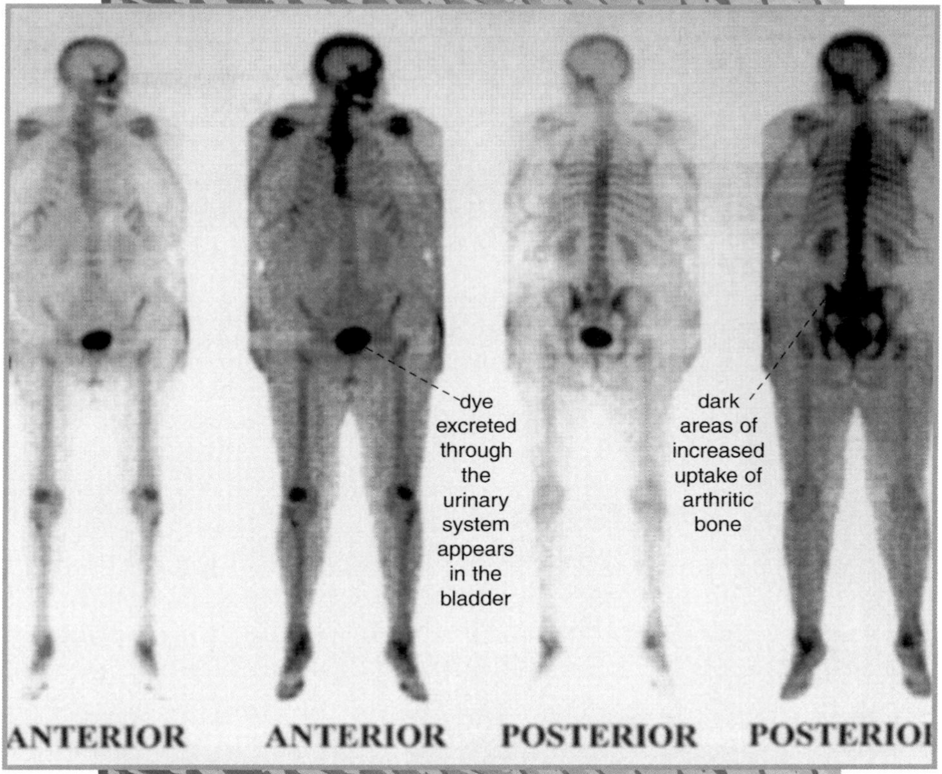

FIG. 5-5. Bone scan showing arthritic bone (dark areas, caused by increased uptake of intravenous dye).

FUNCTIONAL TESTS

Tests of function primarily assess nerve root function. Functional tests are used to evaluate certain patient conditions prior to surgery. For example, if a patient is about to undergo a multilevel vertebral fusion with metal plating on the spine, the physician may need to know how much pre-existing nerve damage is present. This is important so that damage prior to surgery can be considered in evaluating any damage which may occur after surgery. Such documentation can guide the surgeon during the

Electrodiagnostic studies provide immediate information about neuromuscular disorders.

procedure, minimizing patient risk. It also helps give the patient realistic expectations as to whether or not there will be any neurological impairment after the operation.

Electrodiagnostic tests use a volt meter to evaluate the speed of nerve conduction or the quality of electrical activity as an indication of the integrity of a nerve. Such studies are useful in evaluating suspected cases of nerve entrapment, radiculopathy, peripheral neuropathies, and compression syndromes. Electromyography (EMG) tests motor nerves, the larger nerves that influence muscle function and movement (Fig. 5-6). Sensory nerves, the nerves that carry information about pain and position, are evaluated by somatosensory evoked potential tests. Electrodiagnostic studies require training and expertise in administration and interpretation. When properly used, they provide immediate information about neuromuscular disorders.

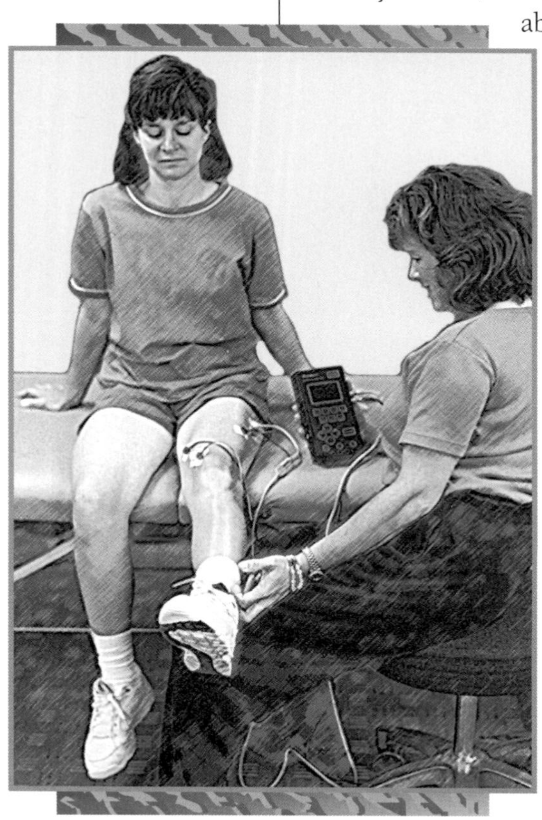

FIG. 5-6. EMG testing.

Although the myelogram and MRI examine anatomy of the spine, spinal cord, and nerve roots, electrical testing is the only widely accepted method to evaluate the physiological function of nerve roots. Physical examination may show evidence consistent with disc herniation in 15-20% of all patients evaluated for back pain, but electrodiagnostic studies can document which patients actually have functional problems caused by the disc.

Thermography

Thermography is another test of function, but unfortunately it is not often used because it is rarely compensated by insurance companies. Thermography involves the identification and analysis of thermal energy patterns using infrared or liquid crystal technology and provides information *not* duplicated by other tests. A thermogram evaluates changes in skin temperature, which is a reflection of blood flow. Thermography is excellent for evaluation of reflex sympathetic dystrophy. We feel thermography holds great promise as a screening and diagnostic tool in neuromuscular and myofascial disorders which currently are diagnosed by physical examination alone.

Ultrasound

Ultrasound has unique real-time capability which permits examination during movement and also allows guidance of block needles. Advances in ultrasound make it a powerful tool for diagnosing abnormalities of soft tissue from the surface of the skin to the surface of the bone. Physicians are seeing more sports-related injuries as exercise becomes more popular. Accurate cross-sectional imaging of muscles can be important in assessment of injuries, and ultrasound can reveal the location and extent of ruptured tendons, damaged muscles, and blood clot. Ultrasound has been underutilized in the United States because of the widespread availability of MRI; however, it is much less expensive and can be performed easily in the office by a well-trained technician.

Diagnostic nerve blocks

Temporarily blocking nerves with local anesthetics and re-evaluating the pain after the block often helps isolate the exact source of the pain.

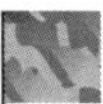

UNDERSTANDING TEST RESULTS

The consequences of ordering a test may be direct or indirect. An indirect consequence is depletion of funds. Insurance companies maintain that there is a reasonable cost for treating a given diagnosis. Thus, the dollars unnecessarily spent on testing mean less funds are available for treatment. Direct consequences are false positive results and false negative results. A **false positive** is an erroneous finding. In other words, the test shows an abnormal finding (positive result), but either no abnormality exists or it has nothing to do with the patient's complaint. The following case study helps explain this point.

Dollars unnecessarily spent on testing mean less funds are available for treatment.

A patient was referred to our office by a neurosurgeon. The neurosurgeon was concerned because the patient complained of upper back pain, and he had ordered an MRI scan. Interpretation of the MRI revealed a high likelihood that a tumor was pressing on a spinal nerve root. The neurosurgeon decided that since the tumor was very small, he did not want to operate right away but wanted to evaluate the rate of the tumor growth. However, he also wanted the patient's pain treated. Re-evaluation of the MRI scan with a consulting radiologist suggested that the shape and location of the tumor was highly unusual for a spinal cord lesion. Because the original scan, done on an older machine, was not conclusive and possibly misleading, it was decided to repeat the MRI in an institution where more current technology was available. The new MRI revealed no evidence of tumor. The first scan showed a tumor—a false positive result. The consequence of this false positive was that for six weeks, both the neurosurgeon and the patient were convinced that she had a spinal cord

false positive: test result that erroneously indicates disease

tumor. More important, treatment could have been initiated based on that false result.

This case also illustrates an example of a **false negative** finding. On the same patient, the repeat MRI revealed a small herniated disc consistent with the patient's pain, which was not noted on the first scan. Not only did the first scan have a false positive, a "tumor" which was really an artifact (an image resulting from the scanning process, not from something present in the patient's body), but it missed a tiny disc abnormality which actually was the cause of the pain, so a false negative occurred as well.

To clarify the downside to ordering a test, consider several articles that appeared in 1994 and 1995 in *Spine Journal*, a benchmark of orthopedic literature. The articles indicated that MRI scans may have a false positive rate as high as 40%. For example, if we stopped everyone who was going to a shopping mall and obtained MRI scans of the lumbar spine, 40% would have positive findings. However, these people may have *no complaints* related to these positive findings. In other words, four out of ten people will have a finding that a physician may say is significant, in that it could cause pain, but they don't complain of any symptoms. On the other hand, the false negative rate with MRI scans was shown to be as high as 27%. This means that about one out of four people will have significant disc abnormalities that will *not* be picked up by the MRI scan. It is important, therefore, to order tests based on the history and physical findings. The ordering physician must have more than a general idea of what he or she expects to see or not see when ordering a test. More information is not always good information; there is a point at which harm is done by ordering tests.

> ***What the physician sees, hears, and feels when examining a patient is the first and most important test.***

false negative: test result that erroneously indicates absence of disease, i.e. fails to detect disease

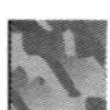

In conclusion, the best test is to look, listen, and touch. What the physician sees, hears, and feels when examining a patient is the first and most important test. At times, physicians need technological confirmation of their impressions, but technology has its limits—it is not the same as eyes, ears, and hands. We should use modern technology appropriately, but the rule is, *order the simplest test which causes the least harm.*

6 Depression: "Is it all in my head?"

For a physician, addressing a patient's psychological issues can be a challenge. It is wise to tread lightly until the patient's trust is gained. We may be the latest in a long line of specialists the patient has consulted. A patient's complaints may have been ignored or misdiagnosed because the specialists he or she has already seen lack a broad understanding of the nature of the problem and appropriate rehabilitation.

Depression can be caused by hormonal responses to pain.

In such cases, depression is common—and understandable. It may take the form of emotional exhaustion and insomnia, magnified by side effects from inappropriate treatment. Losses in work, relationships, and physical function often accompany an injury and contribute to depression.

However, depression also can be caused by hormonal responses to pain. There is no separation between *psyche* (brain) and *soma* (body): the body makes tears when the brain is sad and smiles when the brain is happy; likewise, the brain responds when the body feels pain. Thus, depression in a patient with an injury needs to be treated by addressing the complexities of the problem as a whole and not

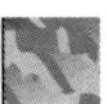

exclusively by psychiatrists or other specialists not actively involved in the rehabilitation process.

ANATOMY OF DEPRESSION

In Chapter 1, we described the neural pathways through which nerves relay information between the central and peripheral nervous systems. In Chapter 2, we discussed the basic anatomy of the spine and the nerve roots that exit between the vertebrae, along with the role of the autonomic nervous system.

The nerve pathway that relays information from the body parts to the brain is called the ascending system; the pathway that relays information back from the brain to the body part is the descending system (see Fig. 1-3). The information is carried by protein substances such as hormones or neuro-peptides as well as other chemical mediators. Some of these substances activate pain; others inhibit pain. The ascending system relays pain through higher concentrations of **pain activators** (mainly Substance P, vasoactive polypeptide, somatostatin, and norepinephrine). The descending path from the brain to the periphery decreases pain through **inhibitors** called enkephalins and endorphins. Enkephalins and endorphins are polypeptides produced in the brain which bind to sites in the brain involved in pain perception. The threshold for pain is increased by this binding action. The important point here is the concept of pain activators and inhibitors, not the exact names of the proteins.

pain activators: substances in the body that increase pain

pain inhibitors: substances in the body that decrease pain (enkephalins and endorphins)

STRESS

A major factor in depression is stress. Stress is the reaction to an abnormal state which disturbs the body's physiological equilibrium. There is good stress and bad stress. Physical exercise, for example, can provide levels of stress that are healthy or unhealthy. By increasing endorphins —hormones that reduce pain—recreational activity like walking or golf can reduce mental fatigue and help reduce blood pressure, body weight, and depression. But too much physical exertion can leave the body exhausted and depleted. In the same way, such activities as listening to music, being with other people, or even sleeping can be sources of good or bad stress (for example, natural sleep is good for the body, but excessive bed rest actually creates unhealthy stress). Poor diet (high in fat and/or alcohol) and poor medication management also cause bad stress by decreasing pain-inhibiting substances in the body and increasing pain-activating substances. All these sources of stress can contribute to depression.

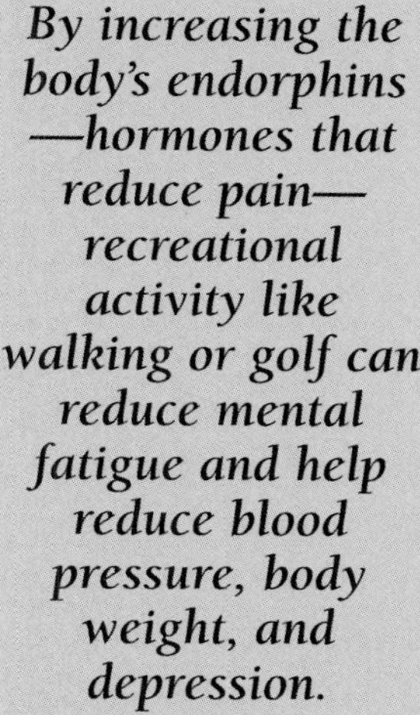

The body is endowed with a complex mechanism for maintaining homeostasis, or balance among its various functions and internal processes. Unfortunately, we don't yet understand all the intricacies of the brain and nervous system that maintain the balance of body systems. With both good and bad stress, hormones are released from brain centers (such as the pituitary gland) and peripheral organs (such as the adrenal gland). These hormones interact to affect the body's homeostasis. Bad stress leaves a person with less ability to cope with pain, anger, or sadness, which may lead to poor sleep patterns and result in depression. Bad stress also leads to pain in two ways: by releasing pain-activating hormones and by exhausting pain-inhibiting hormones. Pain, in turn, exacerbates depression.

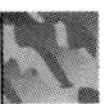

TREATING DEPRESSION

Ideally, patients suffering from depression help themselves by altering their diets to include less fat and more fresh fruits, vegetables, chicken, and fish. Caffeine, alcohol, tobacco, and even red meat and sharp cheese stimulate the production of pain-activating hormones, thus contributing to depression. Short-term use of narcotics, such as codeine, is effective in controlling pain while the patient is involved in active rehabilitation. However, prolonged use of narcotics and sedatives such as Valium, in combination with decreased activity, actually aggravates depression and pain by decreasing pain-inhibiting hormones.

The ideal medication for long-term pain associated with depression is the antidepressant because it raises the concentration of endorphins. In fact, antidepressants can be **analgesics**, or pain-relievers. Because numerous classes of antidepressants are available, physician and patient need to work together to select the correct medication. Some antidepressants have side effects such as impotence, dry mouth, or decreased blood pressure, but usually these resolve after a few weeks. If side effects persist, a different antidepressant should be tried.

Antidepressant medications are also integral in re-establishing sleep patterns after an injury. The body that never rests is on overdrive, which aggravates pain. Antidepressants such as trazodone (Desyrel) help increase healthy sleep.

Society has finally acknowledged that painful personal situations which evoke anger, impatience, and sadness can lead to depression and affect pain. People today are more open to talking about such problems, but the physician must not make the mistake of thinking that "it is all in the patient's head." Talking, whether in groups or one-on-one,

analgesia: reduction of pain sensation without loss of consciousness

may be helpful as an emotional discharge and also as a means of gaining perspective and recognizing that there are choices. The rehabilitation team—administrative staff, technician, nurse, physical therapist, and physician—must be nonjudgmental, centered, and respectful of patient privacy and personal issues. With antidepressant medication, counseling, and physical rehabilitation, patients suffering from depression as well as pain have an excellent opportunity to progress as far as they choose in restoring their health.

PART III
TREATMENT

"I believe that anyone can conquer fear by doing things he fears to do provided he keeps doing them until he gets a record of successful experiences behind him."

Eleanor Roosevelt

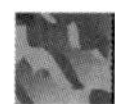

7 Decreasing the Pain

How pain happens in the body—the interaction of the nervous system with the whole body and mind—is an extremely complex subject. These interactions are not thoroughly understood even by the specialists who study them. Indeed, scientists conducting research in the fields of neurology (study of the nervous system) and rehabilitation (restoring normal functioning after trauma) are working at the edge of an important frontier. Although we must recognize that many of the questions we have about how pain happens simply cannot be answered at this time, great strides continue to be made in relieving pain through the combined use of medications, behavioral modifications, injections, and physical therapy.

When patients are referred to the office for a "block," they usually come expecting to receive an injection. However, the term **block** actually refers to modulation of the nervous system at the central or peripheral nerve receptors in an attempt to alter pain perception. Thus a block can be administered by injection, medication, or other means. Blocks can eliminate a pain-causing factor, such as inflammation from a herniated disc, or modulate pain, as in the

block: any means of arresting a nerve sensation

Two major objectives guide the medication management of most patients with chronic nonmalignant pain: enhanced comfort and functional restoration.

case of dorsal column stimulation (discussed below) to alter pain from a permanent nerve root scar. Blocks also facilitate physical rehabilitation by providing analgesia, which enables patients to better tolerate the **manipulation** necessary to correct underlying structural defects.

Two major objectives guide the medication management of most patients with chronic nonmalignant pain: *enhanced comfort* and *functional restoration.* Function includes physical capabilities (if appropriate, the ability to work), psychological intactness (ability to cope with stress), and healthy social interactions. Also, functional restoration should reduce the need for therapeutic care. Ultimately, the goal is relief from unnecessary pain and suffering and increased functional capacity.

INJECTIONS

Epidural steroid injection

Epidural refers to the space surrounding the spinal cord. Steroids are long-acting medications used to reduce inflammation. Thus, epidural injections deposit a low dose of **anti-inflammatory** medication locally at a site adjacent to an inflamed nerve root. As we saw in Chapter 1, such inflammation can be caused by disc herniation, for example, and may result in nerve root compression and altered function that causes pain in the neck, chest, or lower back.

Patients who have had previous spinal surgery may have arachnoiditis (nerve root scar and inflammatory pain), which may respond well to epidural steroids. Epidural steroid injection may also be therapeutic in bony diseases of the spine, such as spinal stenosis (narrowing) or acutely fractured

manipulation: treatment involving direct use of the hands

epidural: space surrounding the dura mater

anti-inflammatory: preventing or reducing inflammation

vertebrae. It also can be effective in decreasing the incidence of spinal surgery and predicting the potential success of the surgery. It is less invasive than surgery because it requires neither a general anesthetic nor hospitalization.

Epidural steroid injection avoids the high levels of steroids in the blood and the systemic side effects that occur with equally potent oral doses of steroids. When the medications are taken orally, they are distributed throughout the body irrespective of specific sites of inflammation. Injection allows for the accurate placement of a minimal dose close to the inflamed site. The three potential complications with this treatment are as follows. (1) The needle may puncture the dura, causing a leak of cerebral spinal fluid that results in a severe spinal headache, lasting from three to ten days. However, this can be treated by plugging the puncture hole with a small amount of the patient's own blood. (2) Epidural hematoma (blood clot around the nerve root) may occur but is extremely rare. The injection should not be given to patients taking blood thinner (e.g., Coumadin). Should symptoms develop (muscle weakness or numbness), the blood clot must be drained surgically. (3) As with any procedure, infection is possible, but with good **sterile surgical technique**, it is unlikely. All medications used are aseptically prepared, and all supplies come in sterilized packaged kits.

Epidural steroid injections are usually done in a series of three, given one week apart. With each injection and appropriate physical therapy, pain will gradually decrease. The block is performed with the patient sitting or lying on the side. The skin over the injection site (neck, chest, or back) is scrubbed with a sterile antiseptic and anesthetized by injecting a local anesthetic with a fine needle. The epidural needle is then advanced slowly. The patient may feel pressure,

sterile surgical technique: operating methods that are free of contamination

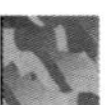

then may feel burning and increased pressure throughout the distribution of the nerve (dermatome) as the solution is injected. The entire procedure only takes a matter of minutes and is performed in the clinic.

Trigger point injections

Trigger point injection with local anesthetic is the optimal treatment for myofascial pain management. First, the local anesthetic 0.5% Xylocaine decreases the pain and allows aggressive manual physical therapy. Xylocaine also deactivates the trigger point by interfering with the muscle contraction mechanism, improves local blood flow, and allows more effective stretch and range of motion. Because the injection temporarily re-creates the pain, it helps the patient understand the concept of referred pain through direct experience.

The actual injection is not nearly as painful as the pain syndrome itself. A fine needle easily punctures the skin, and the patient feels minimal discomfort until the needle penetrates the trigger point. A local twitch response and referral of pain to the involved body part will be felt briefly. Patients adapt quickly to the injections as therapeutic goals are achieved. The local anesthetic acts as a vasodilator, increasing the blood flow to the trigger point and washing out toxic metabolites such as lactic acid.

Peripheral nerve block

The signals carried by nerves are electrical. Peripheral nerve blocks using a combination of steroid and local anesthetic can modulate electrical impulses and thus relieve pain from injured nerves and restore normal electric conductivity.

Neuromas (tumors composed of nerve cells) can form after peripheral nerve injury. The neuroma may be the primary cause of pain by affecting pain-

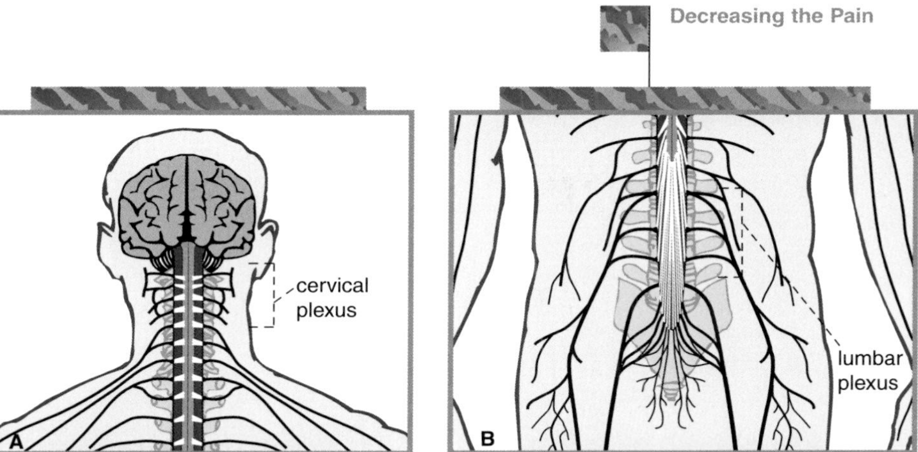

FIG. 7-1. Nerve plexus in A) cervical (neck) area and B) lumbar (lower back) area.

modulating information from the peripheral nerve to the spinal cord. However, most neuromas also have abnormal spontaneous electrical properties in pain fibers, so that mechanical stimulation of the neuroma increases pain by increasing electrical activity. Studies suggest that steroids stabilize membrane conductivity of electrical impulses, and local anesthetics reduce the spontaneous electrical activity.

The nerve block procedure is simple. The painful site is identified, and the skin is scrubbed with an antiseptic. A fine needle is inserted near the nerve site, and paresthesia, or a "shock" impulse, is elicited. Then a combination of steroid and local anesthetic is injected. Associated changes may occur over time in the dorsal root ganglion (sensory relay station of the spinal cord), which also may display spontaneous activity that stimulates pain fibers.

Plexus Anesthesia

Local anesthetic blocks to the plexus (major nerves) of the upper and lower extremities (Fig. 7-1) have been used for years to provide anesthesia for surgical procedures on the arm and leg. In rehabilitation, plexus blocks are used to temporarily eliminate pain and facilitate aggressive manipulation

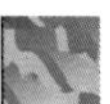

of an injured limb. For example, with plexus anesthesia, patient discomfort is minimal during mobilization of a "frozen" shoulder joint (adhesive capsulitis). Release of joint scar and resultant restoration of full range of motion may be achieved more quickly because the patient can tolerate the manipulations, without compensatory guarding to avoid pain.

The brachial plexus (major nerves of the arm) can be blocked by depositing local anesthetic through a block needle after identifying the nerves in the neck or under the arm. The lumbar plexus (major nerves of the leg) can readily be blocked by depositing local anesthetic via the spinal canal. Pharmacological properties and concentrations of the local anesthetics determine the duration and intensity of the block.

Sympathetic Ganglion Nerve Block

Sympathetically mediated pain involves complicated syndromes which occur when the **sympathetic** component of the autonomic nervous system is dysfunctional. Symptoms usually include limb swelling, changes in skin color and texture, and severe hypersensitivity to touch. Typically, such syndromes occur after blunt trauma to an arm or leg or after organ damage such as a heart attack. Research data clearly show the effectiveness of early intervention with sympathetic ganglion nerve blocks. The sympathetic block seems to interrupt and reset the autonomic nervous system, and the resultant analgesia permits more aggressive rehabilitation.

Lumbar (lower extremity) sympathetic blocks can be performed by blocking the lumbar sympathetic nerve plexus directly or through the epidural route using a low concentration of local anesthetic. Cervical (upper extremity) sympathetic blocks are performed by anesthetizing the stellate ganglion, which is located

sympathetic and parasympathetic: aspects of the autonomic nervous system that work in opposition to each other to increase or decrease heart rate, contract or dilate blood vessels, etc.

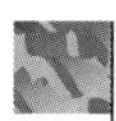

at the base of the front of the neck. A low concentration of local anesthetic is injected through a specially designed block needle. Side effects include temporary lid droop and redness of the eye, which help confirm the needle placement. In addition, hoarse voice, increased temperature on the side of the face and the arm injected, as well as decreased sweating in the same areas, are also observed. If administered early in the course of sympathetically mediated pain, even a single block can permanently relieve pain. Usually, however, sympathetic blocks must be repeated daily or every other day until the pain is controlled.

ORAL MEDICATION

An optimal analgesic medication provides pain relief with minimal side effects. It should be nonaddicting. Ideally, a good medication should not cause tolerance, which means that higher and higher doses are required for pain relief. Also, chronic use should not change the drug's potency.

A good medication provides pain relief with minimal side effects.

Unfortunately, the ideal drug is not yet available. Just as body structure affects body function, so too the chemical structure of the medication affects its ability to modulate pain. Medications currently are designed to function as agonists, which elicit the desired effect, or antagonists, which block unwanted side effects. Combinations of drugs can control pain while reducing side effects. Each drug is targeted to different nerve receptors, and thus each is effective through different physical mechanisms.

OPIOIDS

Systemic opioids (narcotics) act at different levels of the nervous system to take away pain. At the spinal cord level, they inhibit transmission of painful input from the periphery of the body by blocking the effects

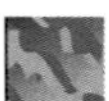

of neurotransmitters. In the brain, at the basal ganglia, opioids activate descending inhibitory systems that modulate peripheral pain input at the spinal cord level. By acting on the thalamus in the brain (the emotional center, as well as the center for processing all sensory stimuli), opioids also alter mood, making pain more bearable. There is also evidence that opioids act on peripheral nerves to stop the sensitization of these nerves to ongoing painful stimuli.

Of all oral medications, opioids have the greatest potency in relieving pain. However, patients can develop tolerance, so that over time, higher doses are required to obtain the same results. With increased dosage, side effects such as nausea, constipation, confusion, and drowsiness are intensified. Regardless of its effect on the pain, opioid treatment is not a useful approach if it exacerbates pain-related disability or undermines the efficacy of rehabilitative efforts. For patients with cancer, many of the side effects can be decreased by giving the drug in the spine via a catheter. By combining opioids with adjunctive medications which decrease side effects, less opioid medication may be necessary for pain relief. The ideal opioid would work at receptor sites that enhance pain relief and not at the receptor sites that cause side effects. Specific receptor sites have been identified for each of these side effects.

The prescribing of opioids and other controlled drugs is scrutinized by federal and state law enforcement agencies. Because of drug abuse, the need to oversee prescribing is undeniable. However, the impact of regulatory policies can contribute to the undertreatment of patients who are clearly candidates for opioid therapies, such as those with cancer. Physicians need to accept the necessity of regulation but also continue to use legally controlled drugs by adhering to current standards of care. At the same time, an effective physical rehabilitation process with a supportive staff can often replace or decrease the need for opioid medications. Long-term exposure to an opioid can create an addiction disorder more severe than the chronic pain which justified the original therapy. However, in chronic pain patients the incidence of addiction (in which withdrawal causes physiological symptoms) is extremely low. This should not be confused with dependence upon the opioid for pain relief effects.

Antidepressants

Controlled studies report that antidepressants can be used to treat chronic pain as well as depression. Antidepressants are effective in treating migraine headache, tension (myofascial) headache, low back pain, diabetic neuropathy, arthritic joint pain, temporomandibular joint (TMJ) pain, and atypical facial pain. As discussed in Chapter 6, antidepressants seem to correct central biochemical abnormalities that occur with chronic pain. Patients with pain who have not been depressed have been shown to have pain relief from antidepressants as well. It is hypothesized that antidepressant analgesia occurs through modulation of pain transmission in the nervous system.

Antidepressants can be effective in treating chronic pain.

Recent studies present no strong evidence that one antidepressant works significantly better than another. There are many different classes of antidepressants; some are sedating and are recommended for agitated patients who need smoother sleep, while nonsedating forms can be used if energy is low. Often antidepressants can be effective at subtherapeutic doses.

Side effects from antidepressants vary widely. Before starting treatment, patients should be told about the most common ones, which include fatigue, dry mouth, diarrhea, constipation, and both high and

low blood pressure. Side effects can be minimized by gradually increasing the dose to therapeutic levels or, if necessary, by switching to a different medication. Within three weeks, many side effects will decrease or disappear. Fatigue should wear off by the third day. Dry mouth and constipation may not wear off but may be minor problems compared to depression and pain. Sugarless gum may be used for dry mouth, and bulk fiber preparations can ease constipation. Standing up slowly can help reduce low blood pressure side effects. Antidepressants have been particularly effective in relieving pain from diabetic neuropathy and postherpetic neuralgia, a chronic pain syndrome which may occur after shingles.

Pharmacology of Antidepressant Medications

Chemical Class/ Generic Name	Brand Name	Therapeutic Dosage Range (mg/day)1	Average (Range) of Elimination Half-Lives (Hours)	Range ofAverage Wholesale Price for 30-day Supply
Tricyclics				
amitriptyline	Elavil	75-300	24 (16-46)	*$0.99 - $4.25
desipramine	Norpramin	75-300	18 (12-50)	*$5.13 - $20.53
doxepin	Sinequan	75-300	17(10-47)	*$2.50 - $15.95
imipramine	Tofranil	75-300	22 (12-34)	*$1.68 - $4.21
nortriptyline	Pamelor	40-200	26 (18-88)	*$17.77 - $51.94
protriptyline	Vivactil	20-60	76 (54-124)	$40.42 - $121.25
trimipramine	Surmontil	75-300	12 (8-30)	$56.69 - $134.87
Heterocyclics				
amoxapine	Asendin	100-600	10 (8-14)	$60.70 - $364.21
bupropion	Wellbutrin	225-450	14 (8-24)	<$50.66 - $101.40
maprotiline	Ludiomil	100-225	43 (27-58)	$39.37 - $81.09
nefazodone	Serzone	200-600	17 (11-24)	<$24.94 - $74.83
trazodone	Desyrel	150-600	8 (4-14)	*$6.34 - $20.05
venlafaxine	Effexor	75-375	8 (5-11)	<$29.98 - $149.91
Selective Serotonin Reuptake Inhibitors				
fluoxetine	Prozac	10-40	168 (72-360)	<$64.39 - $132.08
paroxetine	Paxil	20-50	24 (3-65)	<$56.97 - $142.43
sertraline	Zoloft	50-150	24 (10-30)	<$60.66 - $181.98
Monoamine Oxidase Inhibitors				
phenelzine	Nardil	45-90	2 (1.5-4.0)	$34.50 - $68.99
tranylcypromine	Parnate	20-60	2 (1.5-3.0)	$27.48 - $82.44

1 Individualization of dose on basis of clinical response is more important that strict adherence to dosage recommendations.
* Maximum Allowable Cost (MAC) for generic medication.
< Drug is less expensive than price listed due to volume discounts.
Boldface indicates generic availability. Source: Depression Guidelines Panel, AHCPR, 1993

NSAIDs

Nonsteroidal anti-inflammatory drugs (NSAIDs) act both centrally and peripherally. Because the effects of NSAIDs are unpredictable, therapeutic trials should be attempted to find the most effective agent for each individual patient.

NSAIDs can cause fluid retention, but it is usually mild. They also can cause allergic reactions such as hives, wheezing, and tearing. Most NSAIDs can produce renal dysfunction, so they should be avoided in people with kidney problems. Peptic ulcer and gastric bleeding have been reported with most NSAIDs, and since these medicines also may interfere

Side Effect Profiles of Antidepressant Medication

Drug		Side Effect						
Brand Name	Generic Name	Central Nervous System			Cardiovascular		Other	
		Anti-cholinergic[1]	Drowsiness	Insomnia/ Agitation	Orthostatic Hypotension	Cardiac Arrhythmia	Gastrointestinal Distress	Weight Gain (Over 6kg)
Elavil	amitriptyline	4+	4+	0	4+	3+	0	4+
Norpramin	despramine	1+	1+	1+	2+	2+	0	1+
Sinequan	doxepin	3+	4+	0	2+	2+	0	3+
Tofranil	imipramine	3+	3+	1+	4+	3+	1+	3+
Pamelor	nortriptyline	1+	1+	0	2+	2+	0	1+
Asendin	amoxapine	2+	2+	2+	2+	3+	0	1+
Ludiomil	mapotiline	2+	4+	0	0	1+	0	2+
Desyrel	trazodone	0	4+	0	1+	1+	1+	1+
Serzone	nefazodone	0	2+	0	1+	0	1+	0
Effexor	veniafaxine	0	0	2+	0	0	3+	0
Wellbutrin	bupropion	0	0	2+	0	1+	1+	0
Prozac	fluoxetine	0	0	2+	0	0	3+	0
Paxil	paroxetine	0	0	2+	0	0	3+	0
Zoloft	sertraline	0	0	2+	0	0	3+	0
Parnate	monoamine oxidase inhibitors (MAOI)	1+	1+	2+	2+	0	1+	2+

0=Absent or Rare ◄——► 4+=Relatively Common

[1]Dry mouth, blurred vision, urinary hesitancy, constipation.

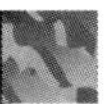

with normal blood clotting, it may be necessary to discontinue them before surgery. Mild abnormalities of liver function can occur, but are usually not significant. Central nervous system side effects include headache, dizziness, and confusion. Thus, these drugs must be used cautiously in the elderly.

NSAIDs are often underutilized in the management of cancer pain. They are particularly effective in relieving moderate to severe pain associated with bony metastases and pain caused by radiation treatment. NSAIDs should be the first drugs used in treatment of arthritis and myofascial injuries. However, since NSAIDs have a ceiling effect, increasing the dose will not increase the pain relief.

Muscle relaxants

Muscle relaxants are medications that act on the central nervous system but have no direct effect on the muscle-nerve junction. They are used in treatment of painful conditions associated with abnormal muscle contraction which can arise from injuries from automobile accidents, falls, sports, or even overstretching. Inflammatory diseases and prolonged, excessive anxiety may create a continuous cycle of muscle spasm. These medications work at higher brain centers and have analgesic and anxiety-relieving properties as well, though the exact mechanism is not understood.

Muscle relaxants also are an alternative choice when antidepressants or NSAIDS may not be tolerated. They are generally nonaddicting, although tolerance can develop with extended use. Drowsiness and depression are frequent side effects, and headaches, dizziness, blurred vision, nausea, and vomiting have been reported as well. Like most medications, muscle relaxants should be discontinued gradually after prolonged use to avoid side effects. In general, muscle relaxants are used for symptomatic treatment over

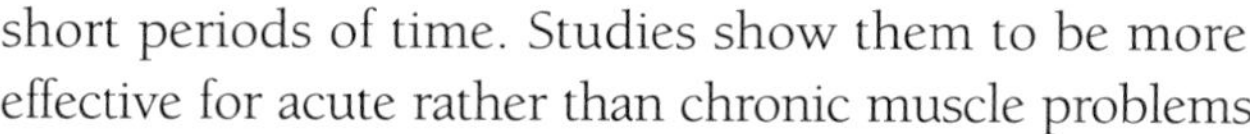

short periods of time. Studies show them to be more effective for acute rather than chronic muscle problems.

Benzodiazepines

Benzodiazepines (Valium is one example) are drugs used to alleviate anxiety and to promote sleep. By reducing anxiety, they have been shown to decrease muscle spasm and therefore decrease pain. Although there are better medications for chronic use, such as antidepressants, the benzodiazepines are clearly prescribed most often.

While these drugs can induce sleep, they typically disrupt normal sleep patterns and thus should be used for the shortest time possible. The most common side effects are drowsiness and memory loss. This class of drug should be used with caution because of tolerance and dependency. Chronic use of both opioids (narcotics) and benzodiazepines (tranquilizers) aggravates pain originating from the central nervous system by depleting the brain's natural endorphin supply. It is recommended that benzodiazepines not be used for more than thirty days.

Chronic use of both narcotics and tranquilizers aggravates pain originating from the central nervous system by depleting the brain's natural endorphin supply.

Anticonvulsants

Anticonvulsants (Tegretol is one example) have been shown to suppress abnormal neural discharges both in the central and the peripheral nervous systems. Anticonvulsants are thought to be effective in diabetic neuropathy, trigeminal neuralgia, and facial pain disorders. Severed or damaged nerves also tend to respond to anticonvulsant treatment. Side effects of these medications, which limit their usefulness, include fatigue, sedation dizziness, weight gain, anemia, nausea, vomiting, double vision, tremor, and hair loss.

Beta blockers

Beta blockers are medications that bind to beta receptors and modulate pain pathways. A beta

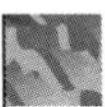

receptor is located in the autonomic nerve pathway and is responsible for modulation of blood flow and heart rate. Migraine headaches and atypical facial pain have been successfully treated with these medications. Possible side effects are low blood pressure, slow heart rate, depression, fatigue, aggravation of asthma, and irregular heart rhythms.

Calcium entry blockers

Calcium entry blockers (Procardia is one example) relax smooth muscles in blood vessels, thus increasing peripheral blood flow by blocking the influx of calcium ions in muscle cells. These medications are used in the management of pain syndromes arising from decreased blood flow caused by overstimulation of the sympathetic nervous system. Since these medications also suppress abnormal calcium conduction in damaged peripheral nerves, they may be effective in treating neuromas and nerve damage from other injuries.

Central alpha receptor blockers

Studies show that stimulation of central alpha receptors, a site of excitation of the autonomic nervous system, can modulate pain pathways. The antihypertensive medication Clonidine is one example of this type. However, the side effects of low blood pressure, insomnia, and depression may preclude its use in certain patients. New information is showing promise for the application of Clonidine at the spinal level to block the critical transmitters of pain.

Peripheral alpha-1 receptor blockers

Peripheral alpha-1 receptor blockers (Minipress, for example) are considered important first-line medications in the treatment of sympathetically mediated pain. Blocking the alpha receptor on vascular smooth muscle causes relaxation of blood vessel muscles and thus increases blood flow. The important side effects are dizziness, low blood pressure, tachycardia (fast heart rate), and impotence.

TOPICAL MEDICATIONS

Topical analgesics have been shown to be most effective in patients with postherpetic neuralgia and diabetic neuropathy. In principle, topical therapies are attractive as an alternative to systemic medication for illnesses like postherpetic neuralgia which involve skin hypersensitivity. Topical therapies are also of interest in the elderly, who frequently cannot tolerate the side effects of oral medications. Often the elderly have major systemic organ diseases, such as congestive heart failure, which prevent them from tolerating oral medications.

CAPSAICIN

Topical capsaicin (Zostrix) alters sensory function in the skin and reduces activation of painful stimuli. Capsaicin is a natural product extracted from pungent red chili peppers. Since ancient times, hot peppers have been used as food additives and as preservatives in herbal medications for pain, itching, and constipation. Interestingly, the medical use of capsaicin dates from the 1940s when Nicholas Jansio, a Hungarian pharmacist, identified the properties of capsaicin and its pain-altering effects on peripheral nerve endings.

In humans, a single treatment with capsaicin produces a temporary burning sensation, which may not be well tolerated. Thus, some patients will not use the cream long enough to get the final effect of analgesia after subsequent treatments. Sparing use of this cream is effective in reduction of pain from small areas of injury located close to the skin.

EMLA

Emla (a mixture of 2.5% Xylocaine and 2.5% prilocaine) is an anesthetic in emulsion cream form

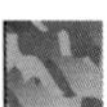

designed to penetrate intact skin and produce pain relief. Emla cream is not long-lasting, and it may take 90 minutes to take effect. However, it may be useful for treatment of minor burns, herpes zoster, and possibly postherpetic neuralgia. Once postherpetic neuralgia is well established, it may not respond to treatment by epidural sympathetic block or peripheral nerve block, and topical agents may become essential in treating the pain.

Studies have shown that Emla produces enough sensory change to decrease the pain of vein puncture, lumbar puncture, and minor skin operations. For the cream to be effective, the body area must be wrapped with plastic food wrap, and patients find this cumbersome. Small pain areas may respond to topical anesthetic cream patches. Improved topical anesthetics hold promise for future treatment of postherpetic neuralgia pain. Side effects are minor. Current uses are primarily to block acute pain such as that associated with needle puncture.

Steroid cream

Nonprescription steroid cream preparations are used as anti-inflammatory medications for local skin rashes.

Mucosal blocks

Since mucosal tissue, which lines the nose, mouth, throat, and other internal passages, is highly vascular, it quickly absorbs medication. For example, the sphenopalatine ganglia (a nerve center, located at the rear of the nasopharynx, which modulates head and facial pain) can be blocked through the nasal mucosa. The block is performed easily by using Q-tips soaked in a local anesthetic solution. The Q-tips are then inserted deep into the nose and left in the mucosal tissue for ten minutes. During this time, the anesthetic is absorbed through the tissue, blocking

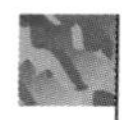

pain signals from the sphenopalatine ganglia. Potential side effects are few, with the exception of nosebleed.

ELECTRICAL INTERFERENCE

TRANSCUTANEOUS ELECTRICAL NERVE STIMULATOR (TENS)

Transcutaneous electrical nerve stimulation (TENS) has been clinically shown to relieve pain. The theory is that TENS impulses transmit at a faster rate than pain-activating electrical impulses from the nerve endings. This electrical stimulation has also been shown to increase enkephalins, pain-inhibiting hormones. For each patient, the ideal frequency must be identified to get the most effective pain relief.

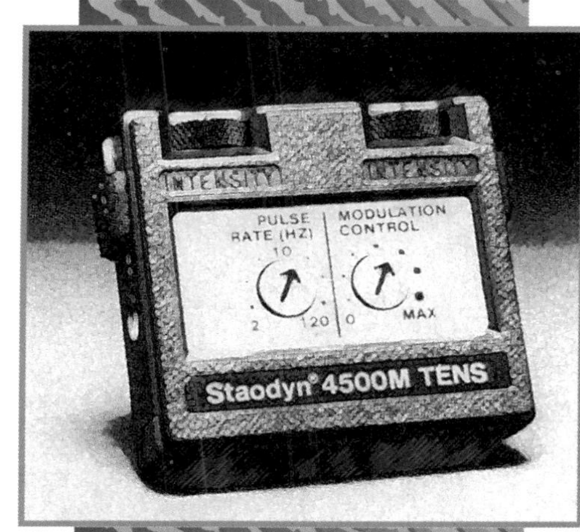

FIG. 7-2. TENS unit.

A TENS unit is a small battery pack with knobs for adjusting intensity (Fig. 7-2). Skin electrodes are applied over the painful area. If the back, for example, cannot be reached by the patient, family members are shown where to place the electrodes.

SPINAL CORD STIMULATOR

A spinal cord stimulation device (Fig. 7-3) is frequently placed in people suffering from failed spinal surgery. Patients with leg pain from peripheral vascular disease and sympathetically mediated pain may also receive pain relief from a spinal cord stimulator. The benefits include good to excellent pain relief in 50-70% of selected patients, with a reduced need for narcotic pain medication and

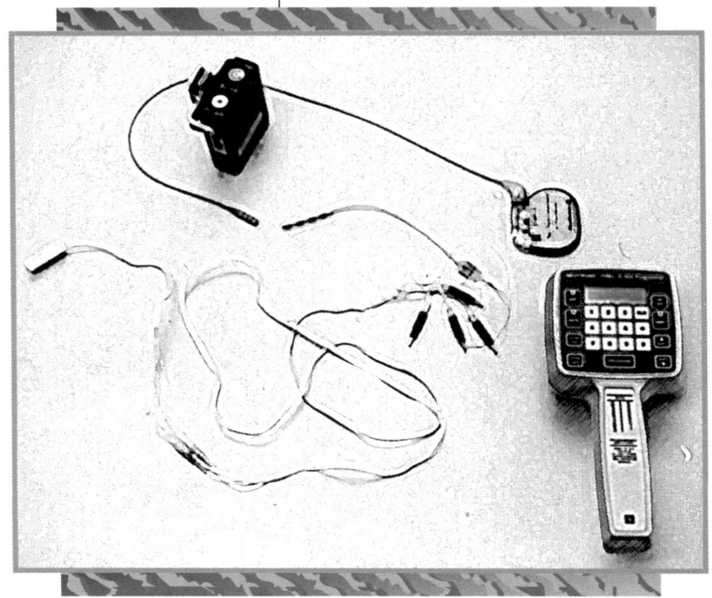

FIG. 7-3. Spinal cord stimulator.

better quality of life. Over the last 20 years, improvements in device technology and implantation techniques make this a viable option for pain management.

The device sends electrical stimulation to a specific level of the spinal cord, which generates a tingling sensation that overrides the patient's pain. It does not cure pain but causes a "busy signal" that interrupts the pain cycle. Initially, patients are given a trial stimulator for three to five days. If good pain relief is achieved, a permanent spinal cord stimulator is implanted.

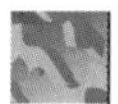

8 Physical Therapy Evaluation

Physical therapists are trained to evaluate the neurological and musculoskeletal system from a structural and functional point of view. They collect information on postural habits used in work, home, and recreational activities; positions which improve symptoms and those which aggravate symptoms are specifically identified. A physical therapy evaluation includes what the therapist hears, sees, and feels, and extensive patient education as well. The evaluation process not only confirms the physician's diagnosis but also establishes a relationship of trust, which is necessary for effective treatment. We consider the physical therapy evaluation a complement to the physician evaluation.

The key to the physical therapy evaluation is finding the foundation of the patient's pain.

Initially, the patient is asked to complete a form explaining the injury. The body outline in Figure 8-1 is used to locate the pain, and the patient is asked to choose from a list of words to describe it: sharp, dull, burning, aching, stabbing, tearing, constant or intermittent. This helps identify the problem and establish therapeutic goals.

The key to the physical therapy evaluation is finding the foundation of the patient's pain. This is analogous to a problem in the foundation of a house

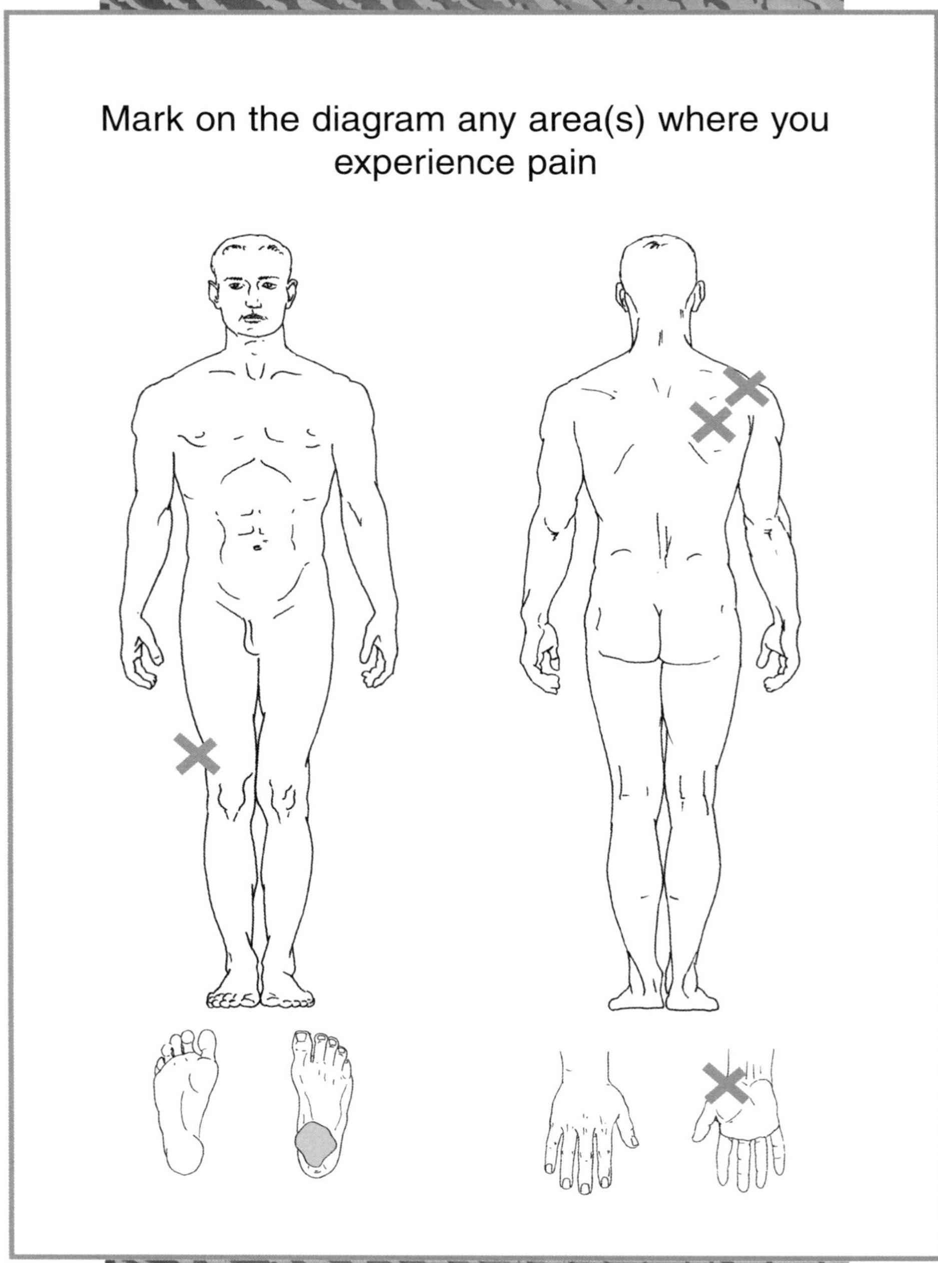

FIG. 8-1. Diagram of body used by patients to indicate location of pain.

causing a crack in the ceiling (Fig. 8-2). The first inclination may be to patch the crack. But the next week, a new crack may appear in a different room. If one continues to patch cracks without addressing the problem in the foundation, the ceiling problem may never be solved. Similarly, to discover the malalignment underlying a particular symptom, it is imperative to evaluate the body as a three-dimensional form, not just from a single perspective.

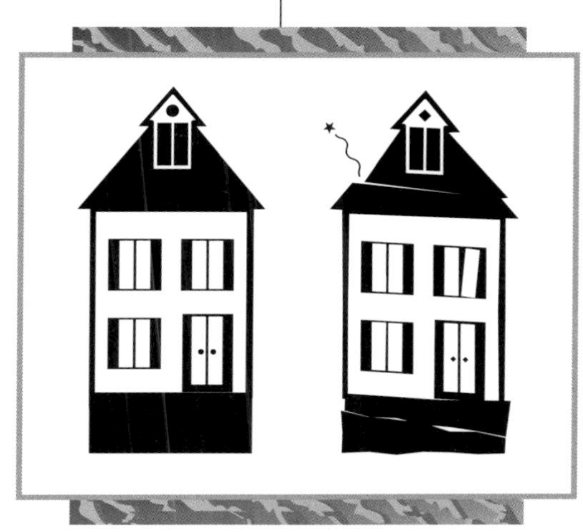

FIG. 8-2. The importance of foundation.

ALIGNMENT

Our physical therapists evaluate all aspects of the body for proper alignment, from the feet up (Fig. 8-3). They first look to see if weight-bearing is balanced on both legs. The hips and shoulders should be level, and the head should be centered on the neck. The body is studied from the front, back, and each side. The normal inward curve at the neck, inward curve at the low

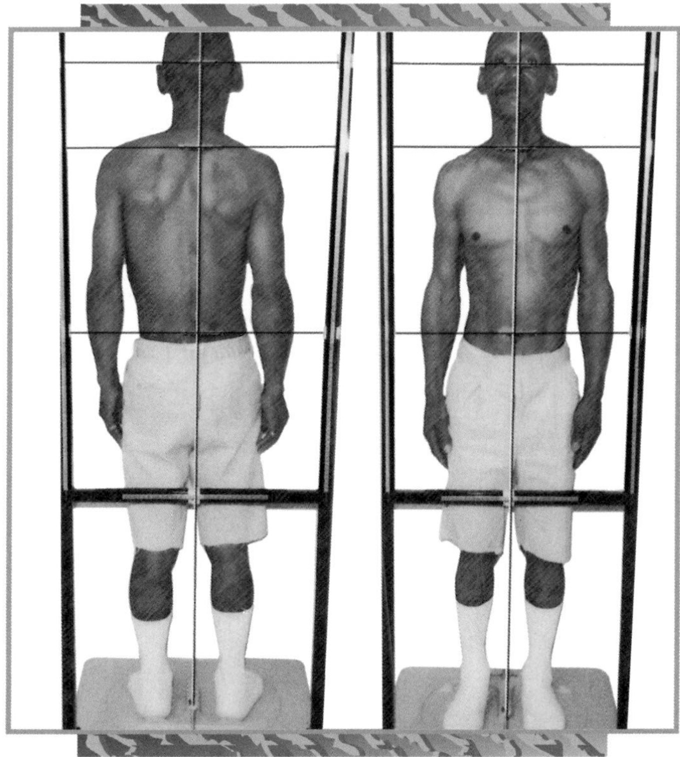

FIG. 8-3. Incorrect body alignment—head, shoulders, and hips should be centered and level.

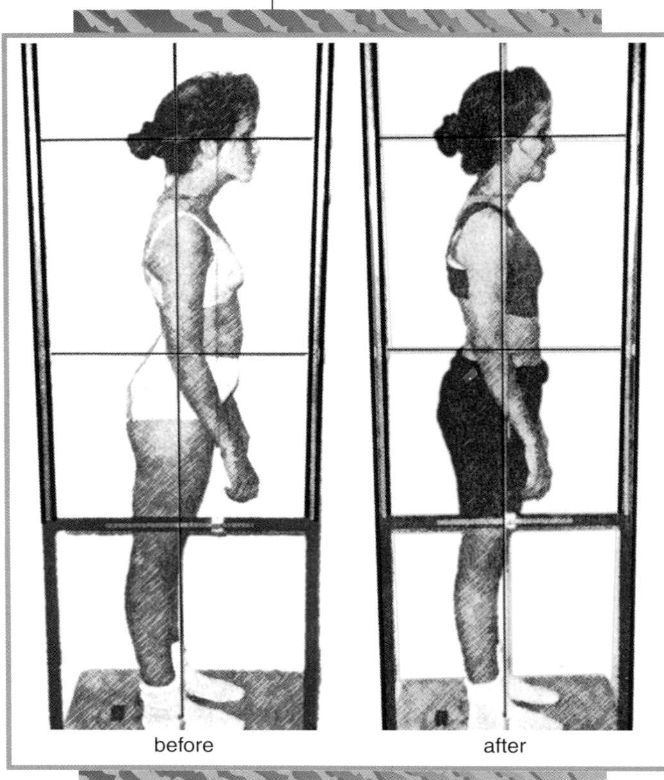

FIG. 8-4. Patient with forward pelvic tilt, causing increased curvature of the low back, excessive strain on upper back, and forward head carriage.

back, and outward curve from the pelvis to the knee cap are checked to make sure no abnormal stress increases or decreases the natural body curves.

When the head is centered over the shoulders, it weighs approximately 12 pounds. For every inch the head projects forward, an additional 10 pounds of force is required to support the head's weight. Forward head carriage predisposes people to pain because the body is not designed to carry a 25- or 30-pound head. Forward head carriage is common because so much of what we do in life seems to be with a forward thrust. When we read or write, for example, the body bends forward, and there is a tendency to get closer and closer to one's work. Except for painting ceilings, not many activities are performed with the neck extended backward. Soon, the body's habit is to stand bent forward at the waist with the head pitched forward and the shoulders rolled toward the front.

Usually, patients are unaware of distortions in body alignment—they simply feel pain.

The patient in Figure 8-4 complained of headaches as well as neck and shoulder pain. Previously, she had had treatment of the neck muscles. However, her primary problem was in the pelvis; both the headaches and the neck pain were secondary to the pelvic distortion. Forces from the front of her body (shortened abdominal muscles) contributed to the forward pelvic tilt. Once the pelvic distortion was corrected, the neck and shoulders could be realigned, and her headaches disappeared.

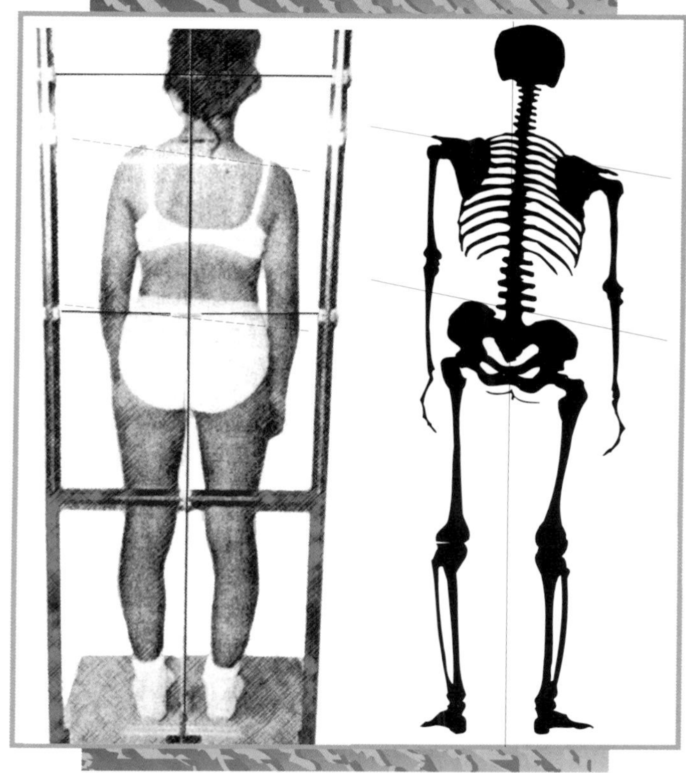

FIG. 8-5. Patient with up-slip of the pelvis (left hip higher than right), causing over-activity of left lower back muscles.

Postural asymmetries such as that seen in Figure 8-5 may worsen over time or after an injury. Usually, patients are unaware of distortions in body alignment—they simply feel pain.

MUSCLE AND JOINT FUNCTION

Muscle length and strength are assessed by various means, and muscle texture and symmetry are evaluated by palpation (touch). For example, trigger points feel like rock-hard knots of tissue, while

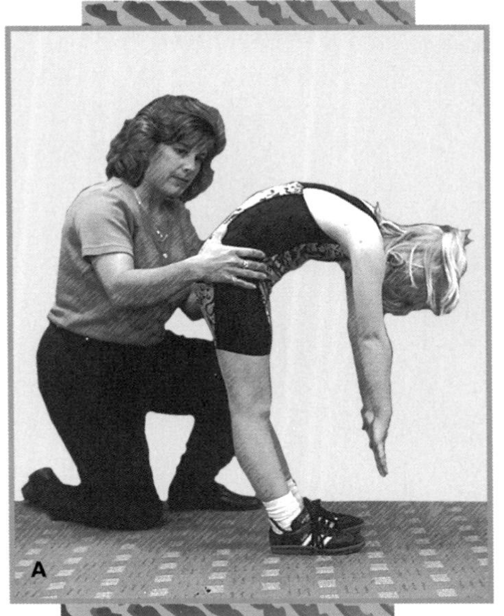

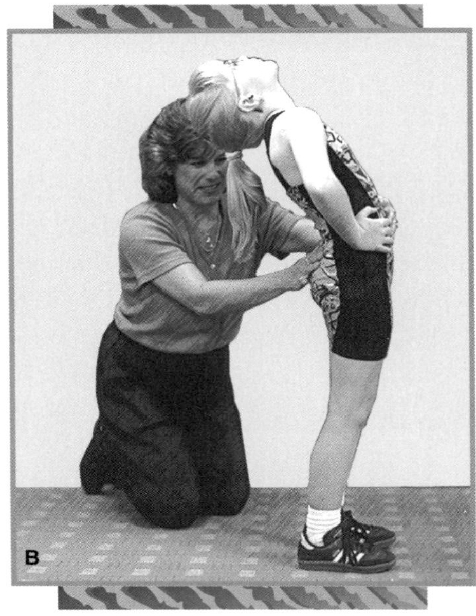

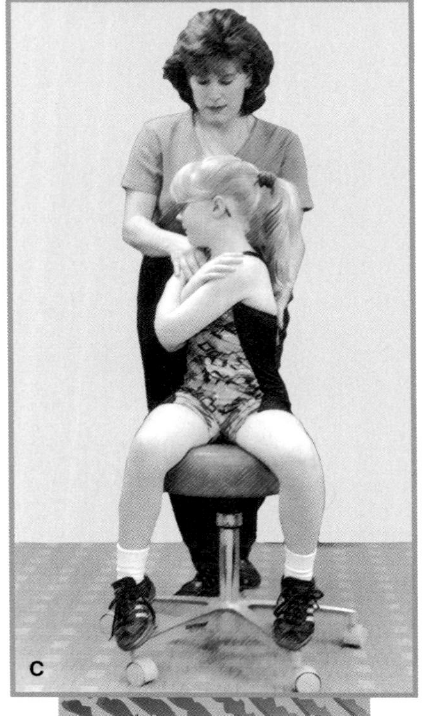

FIG. 8-6. Movements used in evaluating muscle and joint function. A) Flexion, B) extension, C) rotation.

people taking steroid medication for long periods may have muscles that are soft and loose.

Part of the evaluation of the arm, leg, neck, and back muscles involves having the patient perform movements of flexion, extension, and rotation (Fig. 8-6). The range of motion of a joint is measured by goniometry (Fig. 8-7). In addition to the involved joint, major surrounding joints are assessed to determine functional capacity and any adaptive changes that may have occurred to compensate for functional loss caused by the injury.

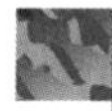

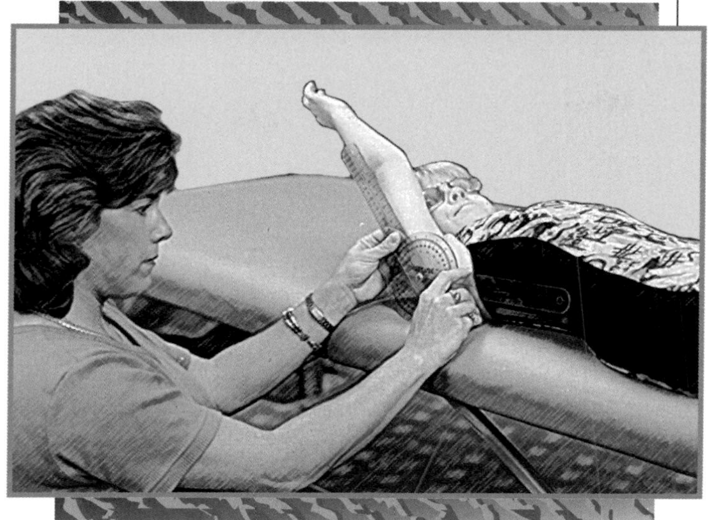

FIG. 8-7. Goniometer used to measure range of motion of shoulder.

GAIT

In the clinic, videotaping gait in walking (Fig. 8-8) can assist the physical therapist and physician in evaluating as well as educating the patient. The therapist checks to see if the heel and foot hit the ground evenly. Is the patient "waddling like a duck" or walking "pigeon-toed"? Each segment of the gait cycle is important. If gait is abnormal, the therapist must identify why some of the muscles are working too hard. Again, the cause of dysfunction is identified.

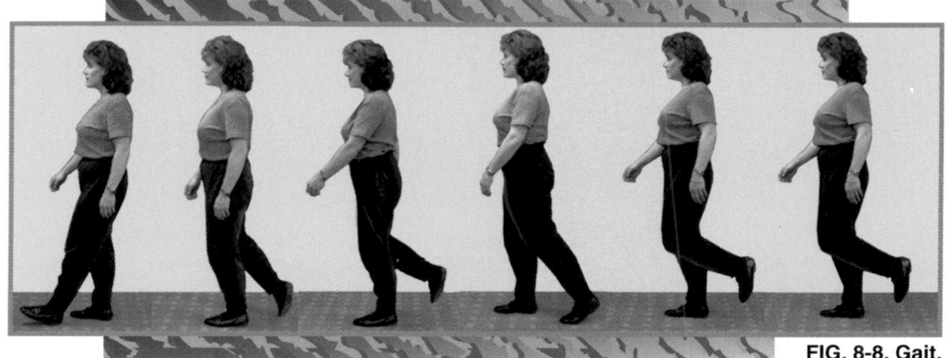

FIG. 8-8. Gait.

STRUCTURAL INTEGRITY

Muscles need to be individually tested through specific movements to see if they are performing their proper functions in the proper sequence.

The physical therapist must also evaluate the integrity of structures. For example, a shoulder evaluation tests for torn muscles and lax ligaments. How far can the shoulder move? Is the shoulder limited by pain alone or by a torn rotator cuff, which may need to be surgically corrected before rehabilitation? How much motion is available in the shoulder in different positions? What is the strength of the shoulder structures? Muscles need to be individually tested through specific movements to see if they are performing their proper functions in the proper sequence.

TREATMENT GOALS

Initially, patients focus almost exclusively on their pain. The bottom line is, patients are concerned about how long they can stand and sit without pain, not about whether their pelvis is level or whether they have full range of motion in a joint. They simply need to feel well enough to work and provide for their families and participate in recreational activities. It is important, though, for patients to understand how their structure correlates with their inability to perform activities. Evaluation is an ongoing process from session to session as the body constantly changes through treatment.

A thorough evaluation includes not only obtaining the correct information but properly assessing that information to make the correct diagnosis and develop an appropriate treatment plan. The treatment plan must take into consideration the functional ability of the patient to adapt. For example, an 85-year-old woman who has had scoliosis for 65 years will never have a straight back like a 20-year-old. But her body structure can be adjusted and balanced to decrease stresses and alleviate pain.

Through patient education, continuing evaluation, and open communication with the health care team, patients can participate actively in their care. In this way, patients share in the responsibility for the rehabilitation process, which is a significant factor in helping them reach their own personal goals.

Evaluation is an ongoing process from session to session as the body constantly changes through treatment.

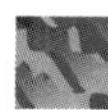

9 The Four Phases of Treatment

Ideally, patients should be evaluated and treated by a physician and physical therapist working together. However, it is commonplace that a physical therapy prescription from a physician often gives no indication as to what the physician has in mind. The physical therapist must start from scratch to develop an individual treatment plan based on the therapist's perspective alone. In our practice the physicians work directly with physical therapists to develop a thorough plan, which is discussed at weekly rounds. Thus, the plan reflects the results of not only the initial evaluation but ongoing re-evaluation as treatment progresses. Like the evaluations by both physician and physical therapist, the treatment plan is likely to be the most comprehensive a patient has had; that is, the whole body is considered, not just the part that is in pain.

"No one plans to fail—they just fail to plan."

Once a patient enters treatment at our clinic, typically he or she sees a physician once a week and has physical therapy twice a week. Physicians and physical therapists consult with each other regularly on how their patients are responding to treatment, and the treatment plan is adjusted accordingly. Different types of blocks may be employed at different stages in a patient's treatment. Just as no patient's problem is exactly like another's, so is there no standard treatment plan or routine healing process. For the sake of simplification, however, we can say that treatment generally progresses through the four stages described below. These are presented here in terms of the physical therapy employed, but the physician continues to work with the patient not only in ongoing evaluation and consultation, but also in administering blocks and prescribing medication to manage pain.

Physical therapists cannot treat a particular problem by following a recipe. Much individualized care, planning, and ongoing re-evaluation are required to carry out a successful therapeutic regimen.

Physical therapists cannot treat a particular problem by following a recipe. Much individualized care, planning, and ongoing re-evaluation are required to carry out a successful therapeutic regimen. Standard treatments such as hot packs, ultrasound, and electrical stimulation may temporarily soothe, but they do not change structural and functional distortion. Physicians and physical therapists must always look, listen, and feel, to develop a comprehensive plan that addresses the specifics of each situation.

PHASE ONE: MANUAL THERAPY TECHNIQUES

myofascial/muscle release: a mobilization technique which emphasizes stretching of soft tissue

muscle energy technique: a mobilization technique using active contraction by the patient to normalize the position of a joint

Myofascial release, muscle energy, and craniosacral techniques are all examples of manual therapy used in conjunction with the blocks described in Chapter 7. Manual therapy is a "hands-on" approach—literally, working with the therapist's hands on the patient. Manual releases are performed with the patient in different positions, depending on the body part involved. In myofascial release, because the fascia is very strong, pressure from the hands must be prolonged over several minutes to achieve lasting structural changes. Muscle energy, a technique in which the patient contracts then relaxes a muscle, elongates muscles and increases range of motion. Recently, because so many people suffer from temporomandibular joint (TMJ) syndrome, headaches, and facial pain, physicians and therapists have begun to focus on manual therapies for the cranium (bones of the head). Craniosacral therapy is a gentle manual technique which balances cranial-sacral distortion to decrease tension on the nervous system. It is based on two often overlooked facts: 1) the bones of the skull (cranium) are not completely fused and can move slightly, and 2) the skull and the sacrum are connected by the dura, the tough, relatively inelastic tissue that sheaths the brain, spinal cord, and nerve roots. Thus, distortion in the skull or anywhere along the spine can affect the entire structure. Once again, with correction of structure, pain is relieved.

The following figures show manual therapy techniques.

The patient shown in Figure 9-1 is an auto mechanic with a history of neck and upper back

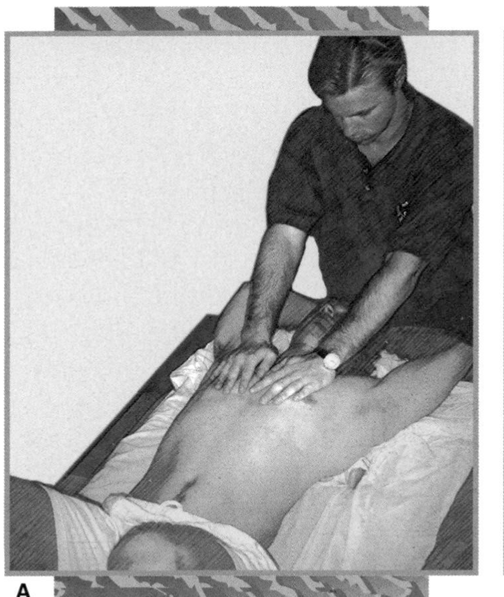

A

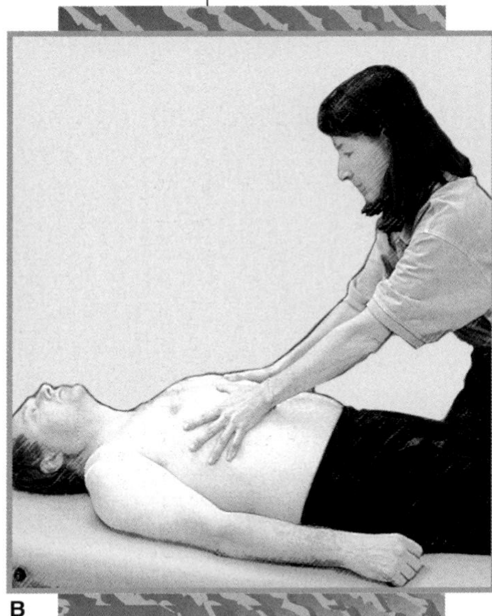

B

FIG. 9-1A. Release of A) front and B) side chest wall muscles.

injuries from an automobile accident. His physical therapy evaluation showed severe forward head carriage and rounded shoulders. He was treated with cervical epidural steroid injections, trigger point injections, and manual therapy. These photos show release of the front and side chest wall muscles which were pulling him forward. Adjusting his head and shoulders decreased the stress on his upper back and neck.

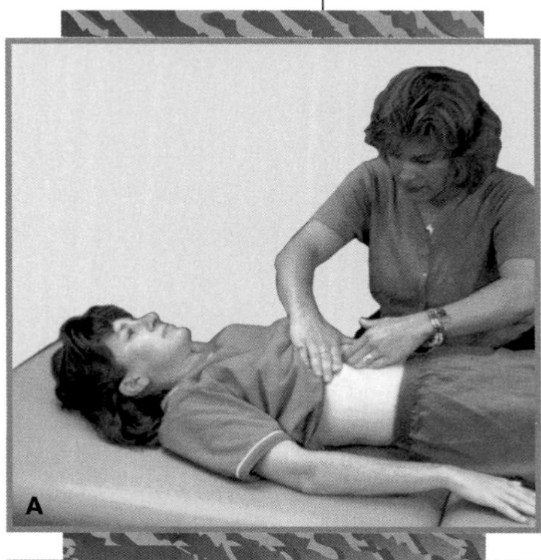

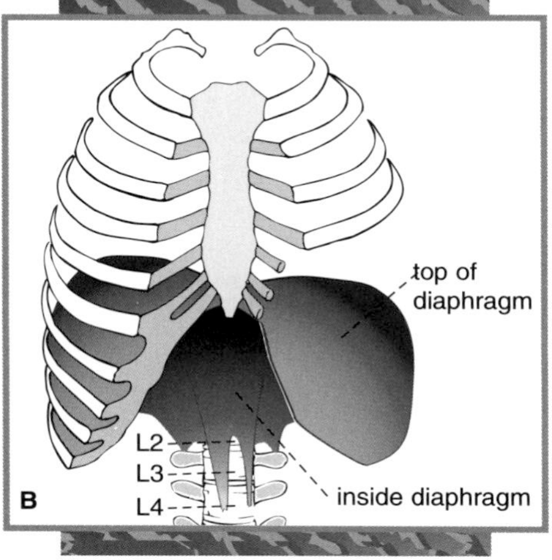

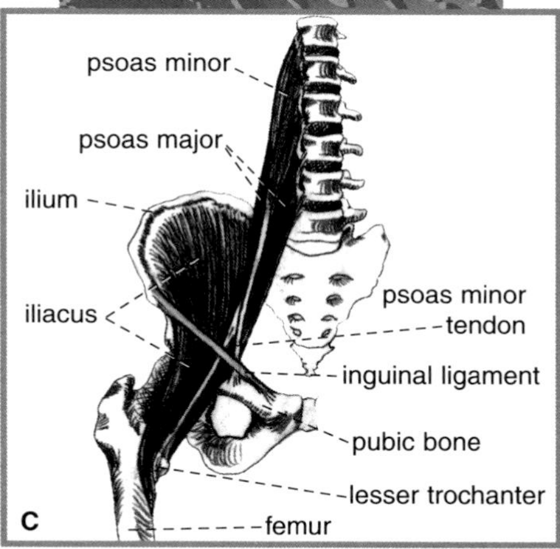

FIG. 9-2. A) Abdominal release. B) Location of diaphragm in abdominal cavity. C) Muscles and bones around abdominal cavity.

Looking at the body three-dimensionally, we can see that the abdominal muscles, such as the psoas, are actually the “front of the back” (Fig. 9-2C). Dysfunction of abdominal musculature causes referred pain to the lower back. Deep abdominal releases are done gradually because this is painful (inducing intense pain can cause reflex contraction and defeat the purpose of the release). The therapist and physician must be patient while working with his/her hands over one body area for several minutes—it may take that long for the connective tissue to release. At times, patients with complicated injuries need two-person techniques to progress at a reasonable rate. With more hands, more of the body can be treated during a session.

A thigh release (Fig. 9-3) can correct shortened inner thigh muscles, which can make a person walk "pigeon-toed." As described in Chapter 8, the therapist checks to see how the foot hits the ground. Thus, the thigh release is important in correcting gait abnormality.

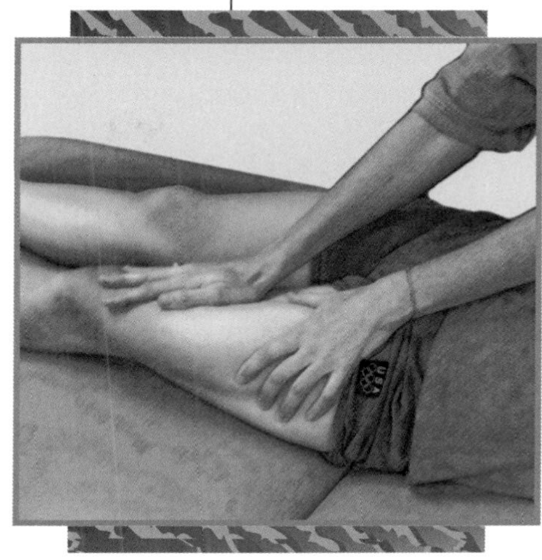

FIG. 9-3. Thigh release.

HOME STRETCHING PROGRAM

Generally, physician and rehabilitation team members teach patients proper stretching techniques from the beginning of their treatment. Not only does stretching lengthen contracted muscles and help eliminate trigger points, it also helps the patient develop body awareness. An important aspect of treatment is helping patients become aware of improper body movements.

Not only does stretching lengthen contracted muscles and help eliminate trigger points, it also helps the patient develop body awareness.

Many times patients say they already know how to stretch—and they are surprised when an entire session may be necessary to teach proper stretch techniques. A stretch is not an exercise; it is a passive movement in a state of total relaxation performed for 45 seconds to one minute. Quality, not quantity, is most important. The patient is taught to stretch until he or she feels mild pain. With each additional stretch, pain lessens as muscles release. The patient should begin stretching gently, setting a goal to increase the range of motion half an inch a day. Eventually, full range of motion can be achieved.

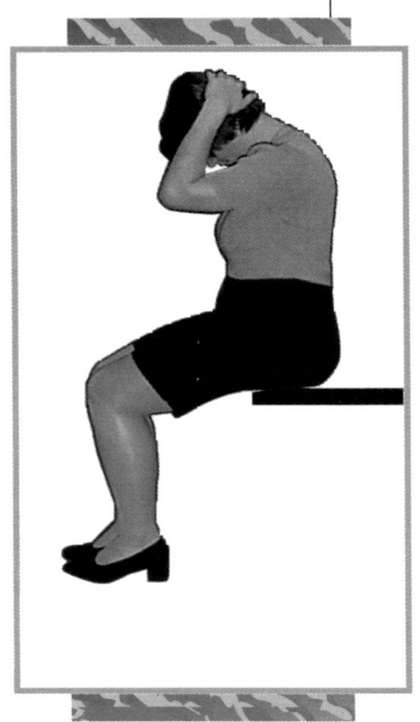

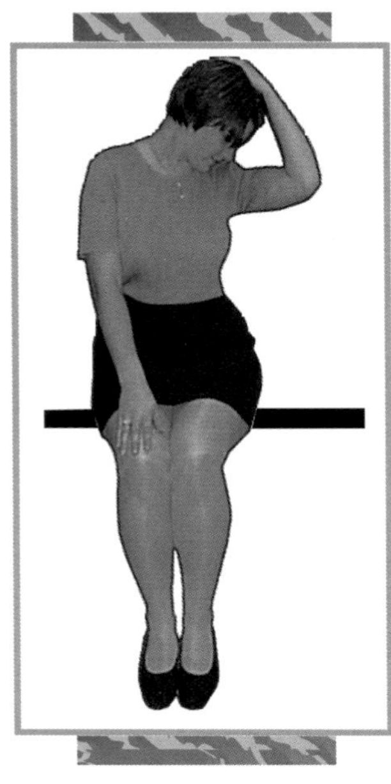

FIG. 9-4. Cervical stretches.

We usually start by giving the patient illustrations of three stretches with written instructions from our own stretch manual (Fig. 9-4). We recommend performing the stretches six to eight times a day because frequent stretching gives muscles feedback to elongate. The muscles stretched should not only be the painful ones but also the ones related to the joint. The patient is also encouraged to stretch during ordinary activities. For example, buttock stretches can be done while sitting drinking coffee, and low back stretches can be done while watching the evening news. Patients' lives should not be interrupted because of a home stretching program—the stretching program should be used to improve their lives.

PHASE TWO: NEUROMUSCULAR RETRAINING

As we have seen, after an injury, poor movement patterns become habitual as the body learns how to avoid pain. To re-establish normal movement patterns, muscles and nerves must be **retrained**. Thus, treatment in this phase begins with isolating and strengthening the correct muscles, then the

retraining: to make proficient with special instruction and practice

muscles are trained to function together. With practice, the brain starts sending the muscles the proper neural messages, and the muscles respond in the proper sequence.

For example, the director of a local health club was treated for severe right shoulder pain and 50% loss of shoulder function following three operations. After completion of phase one of rehabilitation, the patient's pain was reduced by 70%, and his range of motion was almost normal. Re-evaluation of his residual pain revealed he was using his upper shoulder muscles (trapezius) to do all the work and not using his mid-thoracic muscles (rhomboids) at all. In spite of the fact that the patient was an athletic trainer, he was completely unaware of this abnormal movement pattern. He was given exercises to isolate and strengthen the rhomboid muscles, which resulted in greater body awareness and proper movement. Repetition of these exercises, along with cues from the physical therapist, retrained the shoulder muscles to function in the correct sequence. Then the upper shoulder muscles stopped overworking, and much of his pain was relieved.

Patients' lives should not be interrupted because of a home stretching program—the stretching program should be used to improve their lives.

Proprioception is the ability to sense body parts in space. This sense is automatic. Without proprioception, muscles could not be trained to contract in the proper sequence. For example, with your arm pointed overhead, even with your eyes closed, you know exactly where the arm is in space. However, an injury may alter normal proprioception because of compensatory movement patterns developed in response to pain. The nervous system may continue to relay these abnormal movement patterns even after the injury has healed. Thus, complete recovery from an injury must include neuromuscular retraining.

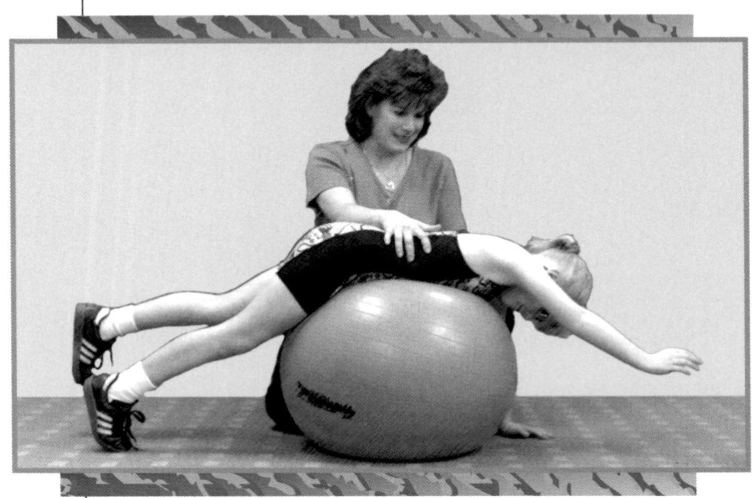

FIG. 9-5. Swiss ball.

Devices used in neuromuscular retraining

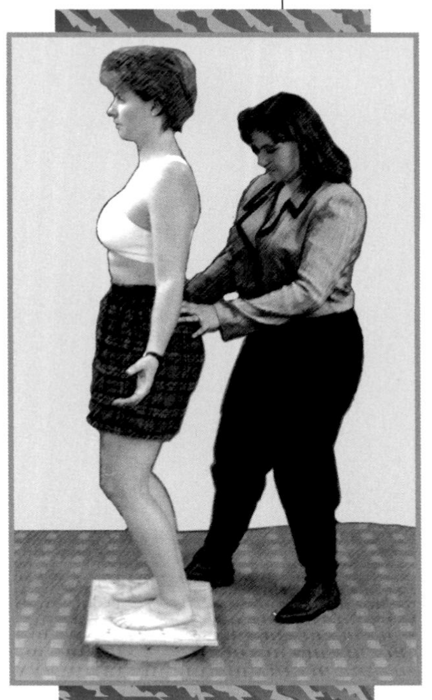

FIG. 9-6. Rocker board.

Pelvic stability is important because it is the foundation of the spine. Usually we start Swiss ball exercises with various movements in the sitting position to isolate pelvic muscle groups (Fig. 9-5). The Swiss ball can also be used to facilitate myofascial release. Working with the Swiss ball can be fun as well as challenging.

The rocker board, another device for retraining the proprioceptive sense, is also an excellent tool for postural retraining (Fig. 9-6). Since it is a moving surface, the patient is challenged to develop quick body reactions. Balance on the rocker board requires synchronized contraction of the buttock, back, abdominal, and shoulder muscles.

Figure 9-7 shows a patient performing postural exercises to stabilize the lower shoulder blade region. Tactile and verbal cues from the therapist stimulate the brain to relearn correct movement.

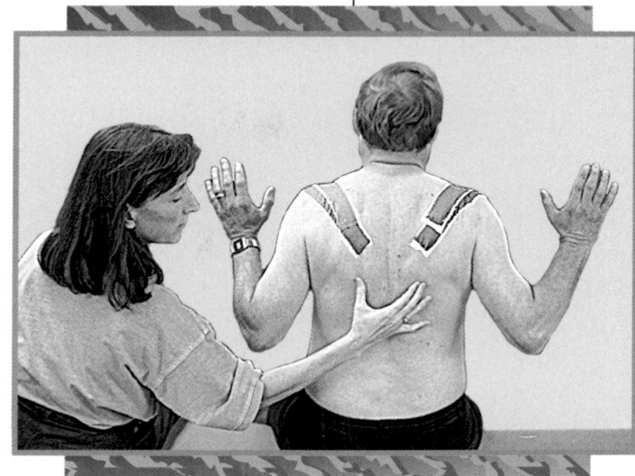

FIG. 9-7. Postural retraining for cervical and shoulder stabilization.

TAPING

For years joint taping has been used by physical therapists and athletic trainers to realign structures and retrain muscles to correctly support the proper alignment.

By taping the shoulder (Fig. 9-8A) in better alignment, for example, the patient can feel proper shoulder joint position and movement. Often patients choose to wear the tape all day since proper alignment relieves stress and feels good. Practice leads to habit; wearing the tape provides continuous feedback from the joint to the brain until it "feels normal." Sometimes muscles that are overworking are taped so those that are underworking will start to contract. Taping, and

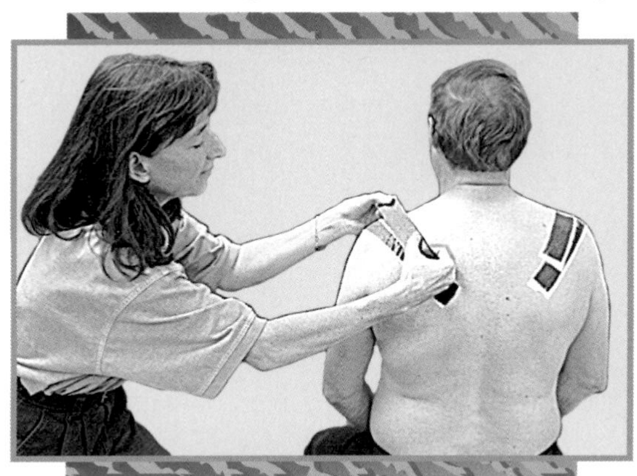

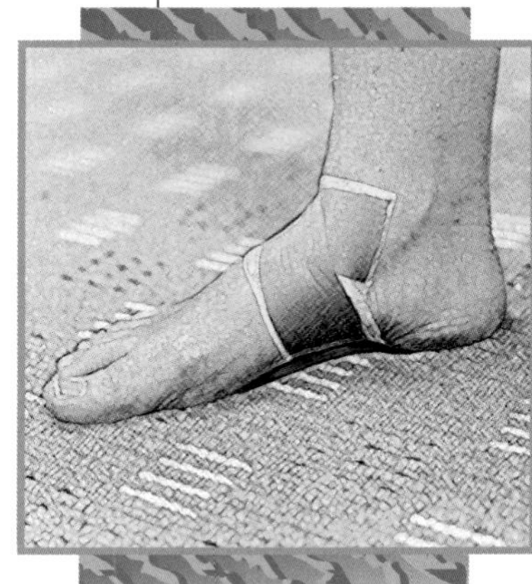

FIG. 9-8. Taping techniques for A) shoulder and B) foot.

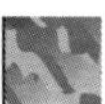

the feedback from taping, helps the patient perform exercises correctly. The tape can be purchased at medical supply stores, and the patient or a family member can be taught proper taping techniques. This way, taping can be used with the home exercise program for postural retraining.

Many patients with low back pain have a foot dysfunction. Simple realignment of the foot may relieve the back pain. Figure 9-8B shows taping to correct flat feet. This correction affects how the foot hits the ground and how the patient bears weight.

Somatic exercises

Once the tissues are released and structures realigned, proper function needs to be restored through retraining. For example, after a shoulder injury, many of the muscles in the lower shoulder blade region stop functioning. The shoulder is then not stabilized as it should be. Somatic exercises involve isolated movements (Fig. 9-9). They may be difficult to learn because the patient doesn't have sufficient movement awareness to move in the required precise ways. The therapist works hands-on with the patient, giving tactile as well as verbal cues until the movement is performed correctly. The emphasis is placed on patient awareness. The patient then practices the learned movement until it becomes a reflex to move correctly. Once learned, the somatic exercises are integrated into the home program.

Many patients have weakness and improper function in the hip and buttock muscles. These muscles must function smoothly in an integrated pattern for normal walking. This is important since walking is an activity we do frequently throughout the day. If the hip and buttock muscles do not function smoothly, the low back muscles and abdominal muscles will overcompensate, creating abnormal movement patterns, and therefore pain.

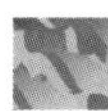

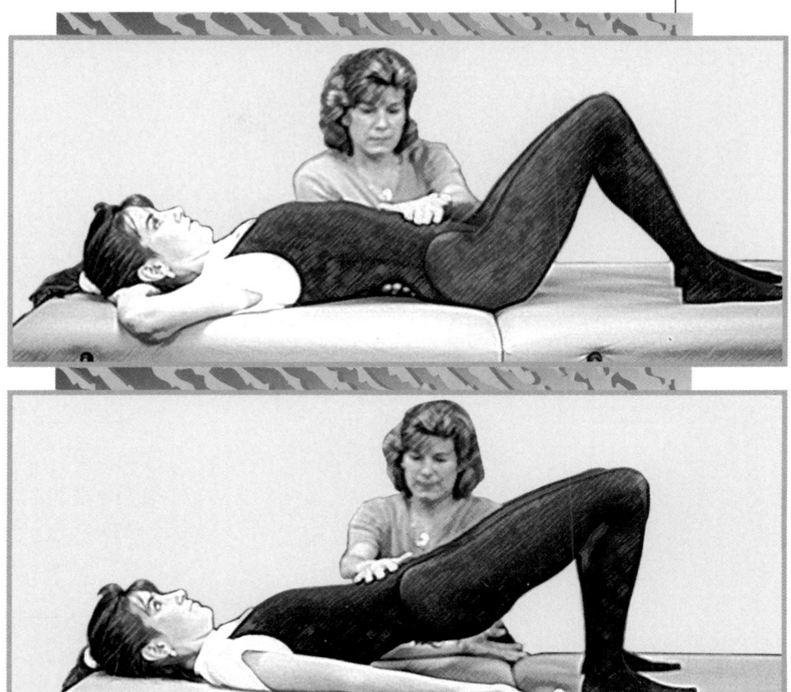

FIG. 9-9. Pelvic stabilization exercises.

PHASE THREE: FUNCTIONAL RETRAINING

Functional retraining begins after pain has been decreased by injections, manual therapy, and medication in phase one; otherwise, the pain reflex that causes muscle spasm and dysfunction will override the ability of the muscle to contract correctly. Phase two must be completed as well: the patient must have learned to contract isolated muscles in a problem area, and the neuromuscular system must be restored so that muscles are activated in the proper sequence. With functional retraining, the patient learns to work the muscles correctly during an

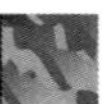

activity. Practice and repetition will make the correct movement a habit.

Biofeedback can also be used for functional retraining. Sensor electrodes are attached to the skin over muscle groups. When the muscles contract, a curve appears on a computer screen. If the patient contracts muscles out of sequence, this will be reflected in an abnormal curve on the screen. Patients get verbal feedback from the therapist as well as visual feedback. A portable biofeedback machine can be rented at low cost so that a patient can work on retraining at home until he/she can consistently produce a normal curve on the screen. It may take some patients several weeks to functionally retrain muscles, and home retraining makes rehabilitation more cost-effective.

PHASE FOUR: CONDITIONING

Conditioning improves the body's ability to function by increasing blood flow to muscles and decreasing heart rate and blood pressure. Any conditioning program is individualized based on the patient's age, anatomy, and goals. Cycling, walking, stairmaster, and swimming are all examples of aerobic conditioning. Aerobic conditioning increases endurance, increases body fat utilization and decreases body fat stores, and elevates endorphin levels, resulting in pain relief and elevated mood.

Muscle tone and strength can be maximized by combining aerobic exercise with a supervised weight-lifting program. Weight training increases the size and strength of muscle fibers, which increases the physical capacity to perform work. The patient may experience 20-40% more strength after two months of weight training. The metabolic rate will also increase, along with an increase in lean muscle mass.

Muscle tone and functional strength are essential for efficient joint function and stabilization. Like aerobic conditioning, weight training increases endorphin release.

Since weight lifting increases muscle contraction, it must be balanced with a stretch in the opposite direction to maintain flexibility and suppleness of the muscles. It is important to remember that an extensive stretching regimen is an essential part of every exercise program.

10 Surgery

Pain relief is important not only to ease a patient's suffering but also to increase a patient's functional ability. Sometimes the only way to resolve pain involves surgery. For a patient who is in the rehabilitation process, a necessary operation must not be delayed. And for a patient who has had surgery, it is just as important that the surgeon make a timely referral to begin rehabilitation. The sooner that appropriate, well-planned, and well-orchestrated rehabilitation is begun after surgery, the better the functional outcome. The best approach is the most complete approach. Rehabilitation specialists working closely with competent surgeons can best facilitate a patient's return to health.

Common problems requiring surgical treatment are outlined below.

INFECTION

Surgery is needed to treat infection or abscess. It is important to immediately incise and drain an abscess to prevent the infection from spreading to other body parts; enzyme reactions caused by infection can destroy tissues. Furthermore, the infection can progress into the bloodstream and even into the

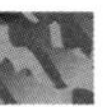

bones, where it causes osteomyelitis, requiring antibiotic treatment lasting several months.

FRACTURES

Complicated fractures caused by major trauma may require surgical realignment of bone for the fractures to heal properly. If bone has punctured the skin, immediate surgery is required for internal fixation of the fracture to minimize infection. Fractures of the spine may need immediate surgical stabilization to prevent neurological damage.

TUMOR

Surgery is required for removal of cancerous tumors. All major organs are susceptible to tumor growth. Also, tumors specific to the spinal cord can affect neurological function.

ANATOMICAL DISRUPTION

With trauma, there may be disruption of anatomy which affects the body's ability to perform. For example, a common basketball injury is a torn rotator cuff, in which major muscles responsible for the movement of the shoulder are torn from their insertion site. A torn rotator cuff, depending on the severity, can limit arm movement, and surgery is needed to repair the tear. Surgical repair is also required for an anterior cruciate ligament tear in the knee, which causes knee instability.

IMPENDING NEUROLOGIC DAMAGE

Surgery may be indicated if there is acute pressure on a nerve, which may lead to permanent neurological damage. For instance, a person may undergo lumbar laminectomy-discectomy if acute nerve compression causes loss of bowel or bladder function or if there is evidence of motor nerve damage such as "foot drop," preventing normal gait. Surgery of the spine may be indicated for spinal stenosis (excess bone caused by arthritis, pinching on the nerve). Additionally, trauma may cause blood clots which can compress a nerve and damage nerve function. These clots need to be drained to prevent further damage. Blood clots in the head (subdural hematomas) are often associated with trauma and may require surgical drainage.

OPERATIONS THAT ALTER NERVE FUNCTION

Some patients suffer permanent nerve damage. In this situation, physical therapy and nerve blocks may not be effective, and surgical procedures such as insertion of a spinal cord stimulator are necessary to alter the pain. A spinal cord stimulator (described in Chapter 7) is prescribed only after other methods have failed to relieve pain adequately.

Surgical procedures performed for cancer pain include insertion of an infusion pump which delivers a continuous amount of narcotic into the epidural space or directly into the spinal fluid. The pump may be permanently implanted if the patient responds well to the temporary epidural narcotic infusion.

Often patients ask, "Why don't we just cut the nerve?" Surgical procedures that cut nerve roots have been advocated in the past to relieve pain. These procedures are not performed regularly today because there can be many complications from cutting, or "transecting," a nerve. A tumor or nerve cyst called a neuroma may form at the nerve incision site.

Neuromas tend to be extremely painful. When a nerve root is cut, the pain from a neuroma may be worse than the original pain syndrome. Also, a transected nerve may intensify pain by altering reflex arcs. Additionally, since some motor nerves (muscle function nerves) are intertwined with sensory nerves (feeling nerves), transection may cause decreased function. Another reason to avoid nerve transection is because scar tissue can develop around the cut nerve, further aggravating the pain.

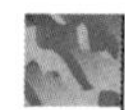

11 After Formal Rehabilitation: Self-Care

When massage therapist Vicki Lander said to us, "I think you need to teach your patients that body care is an ongoing process," we just smiled and shook our heads. It seems that we spend all day repeating over and over again that the body needs care just like hair needs washing and teeth need cleaning. But so often patients want the doctor to simply fix the problem. They expect and even demand it! In those moments, we miss the operating room. As anesthesiologists, we prepared patients physically and emotionally for surgery. When they woke up happy to be alive, and thankful for our part in that, our job was finished. But in rehabilitation, the physician's role includes persuading the patient to take responsibility for continuing after-care.

The body needs ongoing care — just like hair needs washing and teeth need cleaning.

If we were allowed only one word to describe the most important aspect of after-care, it would be *movement.* The body should glide. As Vicki often teaches, "The joints are round and smooth—movement is not linear." In walking forward, for example, the normal pelvis has a natural swing and grace which involves movement in many directions.

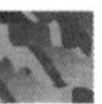

Fortunately, natural, stress-free movement can be learned through various techniques.

It is important to choose an after-care program one enjoys. The program developed by Moshe Feldenkrais—an Israeli physicist who became interested in movement because he was plagued with severe joint pain—teaches movement exercises to increase body awareness. A similar approach is taught in the Alexander method. Joseph Pilates, a German, combined his knowledge of engineering, Zen, and ancient Greek and Roman exercise to develop a movement program. The Pilates method works many of the deeper muscles together, improving coordination and balance to achieve efficient and graceful movement. Much can be gained by dance classes and martial arts such as tai chi, which focus on body awareness and efficient movement. Many community centers teach classes in yoga, stretching, deep breathing, and meditation. Some of our patients have surprised themselves by dedicating precious time to yoga because it makes them feel so great.

Exercise, stretching, and a reasonable lifestyle are necessary to maintain proper structure and function of the body. For those of us with unreasonable lifestyles, regular massage therapy is essential. In our community there are many aware, well-trained massage therapists. We make every effort to encourage our patients to follow-up with massage as necessary.

As we age, life should be richer and more fulfilling. So, take a deep breath, and let it all in.

PART IV
CASE STUDIES

"*The strongest principle of growth lies in human choice.*"

George Eliot

1 Case Study: Headache

HISTORY

A generally healthy 12-year-old boy had been kicked in the left side of the jaw while playing goalie in a soccer game. The injury had occurred one year prior to his Injury Specialists consultation. The impact of the kick was so severe it threw the patient to the ground, causing loss of consciousness for several minutes. Since that time, the patient stated he had daily frontal headaches, which were aggravated by noise and lack of sleep. Before the injury, the patient was a straight-A student and participated in all types of sports. Since the injury, he had missed many days of school and was unable to regularly participate in sports.

The patient saw several different specialists, including those at two major children's hospitals. Of the more than ten different medications prescribed, some provided intermittent relief, but none cured the headaches. He had had two CT scans of the head, which showed no abnormalities. Many consultants had recommended the parents consider pediatric psychiatric counseling for the headache syndrome, which they refused to do. (As the mother said, "This kid was

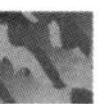

fine until he got kicked in the head, and they're telling me he needs to see a shrink? I don't think so.") Eventually, the patient was referred to Injury Specialists by a pediatric neurologist.

PERTINENT PHYSICAL FINDINGS

Physical examination revealed the patient's left eyebrow to be higher than the right, the left collarbone higher than the right, and the left hip higher than the right. The patient's left foot was internally rotated, making him walk "pigeon-toed" on the left. The muscles of the upper neck and torso on the left side were more contracted than those on the right. This caused an anterior thoracic torsion (twisted chest). The patient's abdomen was rigid, and the diaphragm was severely contracted as well. The patient could turn his head towards the right but had difficulty turning it towards the left.

TREATMENT

For five weeks the patient received trigger point injections (up to eight each week) in the neck muscles. During trigger point injection, the patient could feel the referral of pain from the neck muscles shooting up the back of his head to the front of his head. The patient then had manual myofascial release physical therapy. The low back muscles were released first, and the pelvis was made level. The leg muscles were also released so the patient could walk normally. His diaphragm muscle was released, which enabled him to stand up straight. Eight weeks after the initial treatment, the patient exited from our care. He was able to compete again in sports. He stopped missing school. His headaches were relieved.

DISCUSSION

There are thousands of books written about headache syndromes, and numerous texts describe headaches caused by brain tumors, cerebral aneurysms, and vascular disorders. However, there are also headaches caused by trauma. In this case, the trauma was obvious. Before the soccer injury the patient was extremely active; after the injury he had a chronic headache. When no one could cure the headache, it was suggested the problem was purely emotional. In fact, as this case demonstrates, the problem was structural.

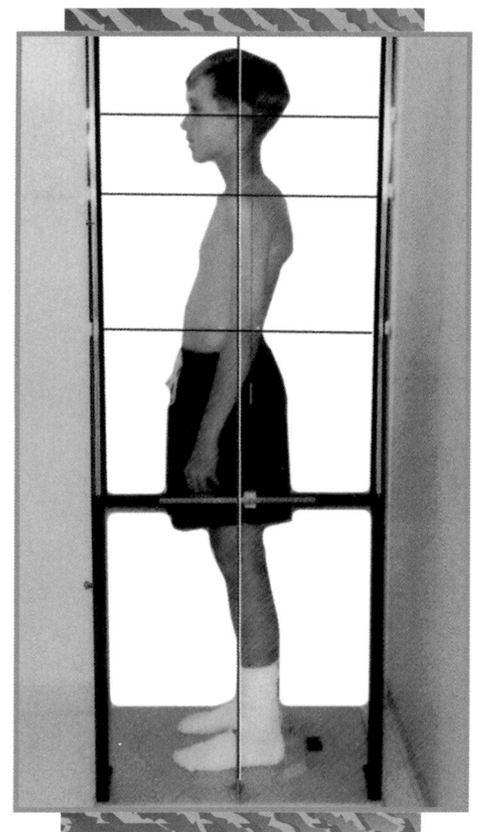

Before

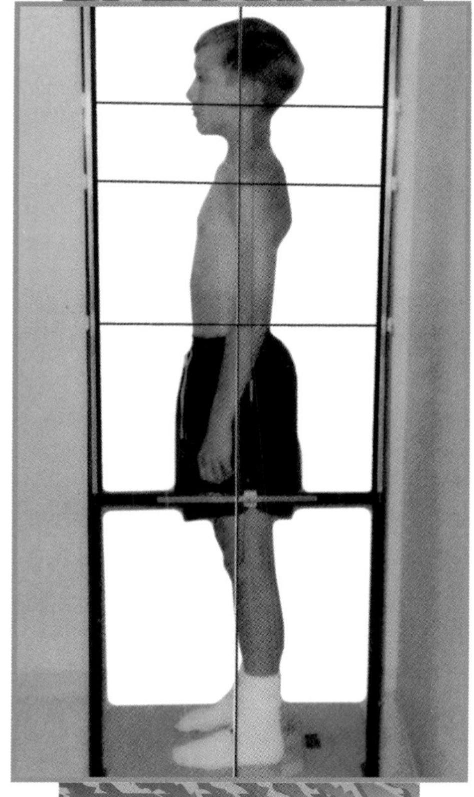

After

2 Case Study: Left Hip Pain

HISTORY

A 56-year-old woman was referred to the office by a respected neurosurgeon. Her chief complaint was a ten-year history of pain radiating from her left hip down her left leg. At times she experienced numbness in her foot. The patient was happily married, worked full-time at a local clothing store, and was very active in spite of her pain. She stated that she had been well until 1985 when she had a neuroma (nerve cyst) removed from her left hip. The patient stated that since then, she had seen neurosurgeons, family practitioners, chiropractic physicians, and physical therapists. In addition to her insurance coverage, she had spent more than $10,000 of her own money seeking relief. Her pain was worse in the morning and was aggravated by sitting, lifting, lying down, and bending. She felt some relief from wearing a girdle and using a heating pad. She stated that her sleep was constantly interrupted and she had given up many recreational activities, such as riding in her motor boat, which she used to love. The patient had been told that her sacrum was fused to the ilium (the lateral pelvic bone).

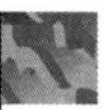

PERTINENT PHYSICAL FINDINGS

Physical examination revealed an appropriately anxious, tearful woman. She could bend forward and touch the floor, but she had minimal movement of her lower spine, which moved as if it were a flat board. When she walked, she favored her left leg because of the pain. The right side of her pelvis was twisted, which made her right leg appear longer than her left leg, though both legs were the same length. Palpation revealed distinct tenderness over the left area of the sacroiliac joint (lower back). She had contraction and sensitivity of the major low back muscle (quadratus lumborum) and of all her buttock muscles (gluteus maximus, medius, and minimus) on the left side, which pulled the left hip up, making the left leg appear shorter. The patient's left sacroiliac joint dysfunction most likely developed after her operation ten years ago, as the patient probably favored the left leg because of pain from the surgical procedure. The body then learned not to move this joint, and subsequently the pain syndrome developed.

TREATMENT

Treatment included two left sacroiliac joint steroid injections performed one week apart. After each injection, the patient was treated with hip scouring and extraction, which are manual decompression techniques. The patient also had three sessions of trigger point injections to the lower left back muscle and gluteal muscles. The combination of trigger point injections and myofascial release physical therapy corrected the pelvic torsion. At the time of discharge, three and a half weeks after the initial evaluation, the patient had a normal, balanced pelvis. She had

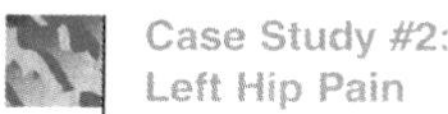

excellent movement. She had been essentially pain-free for over ten days and talked about riding in her motor boat.

DISCUSSION

Although this patient had been told that her ilium was fused to her sacrum, she was not informed that this could be treated with aggressive manual techniques. This case illustrates that it is important to integrate the physical examination and x-ray information for proper diagnosis and rehabilitation treatment.

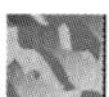

3 Case Study: Back Pain and "Post-Polio Syndrome"

HISTORY

A 39-year-old woman was referred by a prominent neurosurgeon for treatment of back pain. Her complicated history involved polio at age three, with residual left leg and left lower body weakness. Over the years, the patient had compensated for this quite well and worked as a restaurant manager and bartender. At age 13, the patient had Harrington rods inserted for severe scoliosis. At age 24, the patient had surgery to remove the Harrington rods because they were broken. At age 35, four years prior to evaluation by Injury Specialists, the patient had appropriate surgery to remove vertebral bone pressing on spinal nerve roots. This partially relieved her pain, but she still had severe, intractable pain across the lower back, radiating to the right toes. The patient was re-evaluated by the neurosurgeon, who felt no further surgical procedure would be useful. The patient reported to our office with a folder full of x-rays. She had also seen numerous specialists and had been diagnosed with "post-polio syndrome," a pain syndrome which may appear years later as a consequence of polio.

PERTINENT PHYSICAL FINDINGS

Pertinent physical findings revealed a woman with very poor muscle tone. Her spine was almost S-shaped at initial evaluation. She had a long scar from the base of the skull to the base of the spine and no movement in the spine because it had been fused surgically. Her right hip was pulled up, and the muscles on the right side along the spine were severely contracted and very tight. Evaluation of the patient's hip muscles showed no tone in her buttocks at all. The patient's feet were also very flat. Her left leg was much thinner than her right leg; she did not have the same muscle tone and function in her left thigh or left leg because of the polio. She walked with a severe limp in her right leg, forcing her left hip to shift laterally because of weakness in the left leg. The left leg was also externally rotated.

TREATMENT

The first phase of the patient's treatment involved structural correction. During this 12-week period, her pelvis was balanced, her forward head carriage was corrected, and her shoulders were realigned. She was also fitted with an orthotic to provide arch support. Her pain level came down from a constant 10 to a 4 (on a scale of 1-10 with 10 being the worst pain). Towards the end of her treatment, there were several weeks when she did not progress, and we released her from our care. At the time, we felt that she could not improve further because of the residual polio defects and the spinal fusion.

The patient came back for a second round of treatment ten months later. She had been doing her stretches faithfully, and most of the previous structural improvements had remained intact. Meanwhile, through continuing education, the rehabilitation team had learned more about neuromuscular facilitation (getting muscles to work correctly) and had started to work aggressively with techniques which stimulate the nervous system. With our new knowledge of neuromuscular retraining, it became obvious that the reason her buttock muscles were so flaccid was that they were not working.

Muscle testing identified abnormal muscle constriction and inhibiting patterns; for example, the deep abdominal muscles (the "front of the back") were not activating. Because of her spinal fusion, the patient was not treated with aggressive bone manipulation but with soft-tissue manipulation, which "turned on" the nervous system. Muscles which were previously not working started to support her body to work in the proper sequence and at the proper speed. Specific exercises were given to retrain her muscles, and repetition of certain exercises made proper movement a normal reflex. Exercises on the rocker board and the swiss ball along with biofeedback and some body awareness were part of the retraining. Her husband made her a rocker board, and her neuromuscular exercises are now a part of her daily routine. The patient's pain was completely abated on most days, and she stopped all pain medications.

DISCUSSION

At her exit evaluation, the patient's body structure was significantly improved. Obviously, because of the polio and spinal fusion, it was not perfect. However, it was balanced enough for her to have minimal pain. On the patient's last day, she gave a big smile and said, "I finally have buns of steel."

4 Case Study: Pain after a Motor Vehicle Accident

HISTORY

A 13-year-old boy was referred to the office approximately one year after a school bus accident in which the patient was thrown around in the bus, hitting his head on a window. One year later he still had intractable headaches, neck pain, and back pain, along with severe tingling and numbness down his right arm. Because the pain interfered with his concentration, it was difficult for him to complete his school work, and he could not participate in choir or sports. He was evaluated by numerous physicians, including two orthopedic surgeons, a neurologist, a general practitioner, a pediatrician, and an oral surgery specialist. He also was treated with physical therapy for eight weeks. His physical therapy included some soft-tissue mobilization, which changed his pain from a 10 to a 7. However, his pain was still constant, and it was exaggerated by stress, changes in weather, and recreational activities. Fortunately, it did not affect sleep. The patient had x-rays of his head and neck twice and nerve conduction studies, all of which showed no abnormalities. He had been discharged

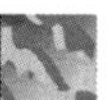

by his previous physical therapist as maximally medically improved. He did not want to try braces as recommended by the oral surgery specialist.

PERTINENT PHYSICAL FINDINGS

The patient had dramatic forward head carriage. Evaluation of his face showed that his left eye appeared much lower than his right eye, and his left neck muscles were severely contracted. This caused left rotation of several neck vertebrae. Palpation of these muscles caused tingling and numbness in his right hand. The right shoulder was elevated and shifted forward, and the pelvis was tilted forward, making the patient's lower back appear swayed. His chest was indented. Palpation of lower back trigger points made the patient's heart race and his skin perspire.

TREATMENT

The above body distortions were individually addressed. The pelvis was balanced with lower back trigger point injections and myofascial release physical therapy. The increased heart rate and skin perspiration abated after the pelvis was balanced. Muscle energy techniques performed over several visits realigned the spine. Intensive myofascial release of chest muscles and neck muscles corrected the forward head carriage. Gradually, the patient's mood went from silent and despondent to talkative, entertaining, and enthusiastic.

DISCUSSION

After eight weeks the patient returned to choir and sports. He was able to resume writing, a personal passion. During choir rehearsal, his voice felt full and relaxed.

Injuries from motor vehicle accidents are often difficult to treat because with pure myofascial pain, diagnostic studies will be negative. Also, patients may wish to pursue litigation and may malinger for a dollar settlement. However, careful history and physical examination can be very specific in identifying malingering patients. This can be a tough and painful process for the rehabilitation team, but is nonetheless a responsibility.

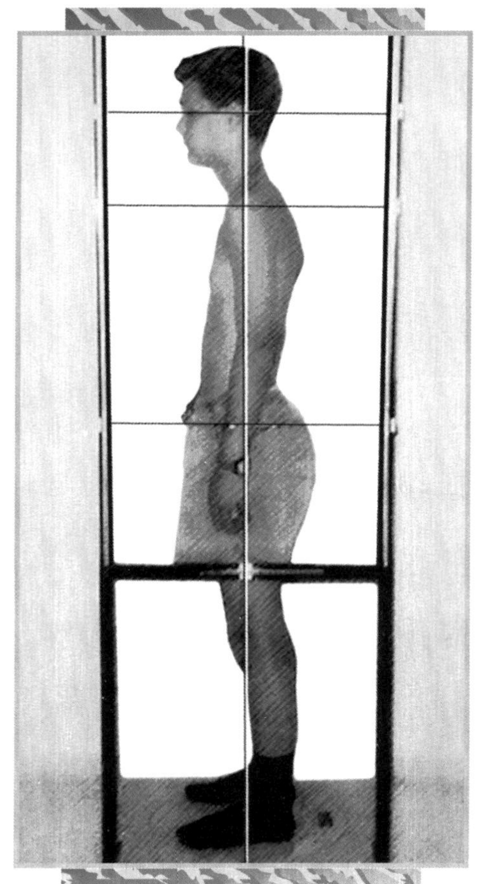

Before

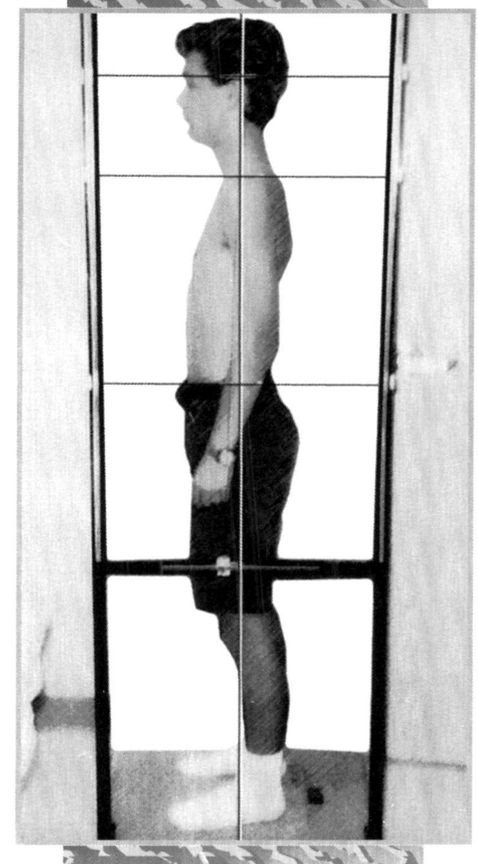

After

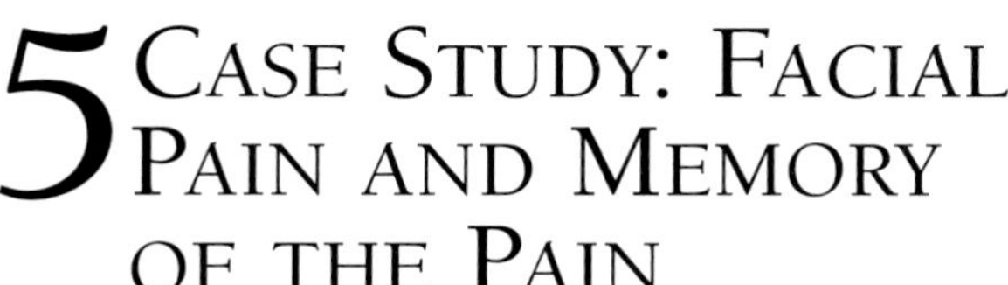

5 Case Study: Facial Pain and Memory of the Pain

HISTORY

This patient was a 56-year-old man who heard us give a lecture on myofascial pain. His chief complaint was pain in the left side of his face, left shoulder, and left front chest. The patient had seen numerous consultants and a dentist who diagnosed temporomandibular joint dysfunction (TMJ). The dentist had been very informative and had shown the patient how to stretch his facial muscles, but the patient still had significant pain.

PERTINENT PHYSICAL FINDINGS

The physical examination revealed the patient's left shoulder to be higher than his right shoulder and the front neck muscles to be very tight. The patient felt constant left chest pressure. He was treated with trigger point injections and aggressive myofascial release physical therapy and was extremely compliant with his home stretching program. His pain level

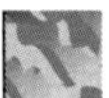

dropped from 10 to 3. After 12 weeks of therapy, the patient stated he was definitely much better, but he still had not achieved his goal. At this point, both the physician and physical therapist considered the patient's body to be well aligned and free from constriction. His chest muscles and shoulder had relaxed, and we did not detect any trigger points.

TREATMENT

We sat and spoke with the patient, asking him if there was anything he could remember about the onset of his pain. He had been giving this a lot of thought. Finally, he recalled several events which occurred the day he first experienced the pain, more than ten years earlier. The patient had quit his job because his new employer was unethical; he recalled the anger and frustration he felt then. On that same day, a close friend of his son's had been found murdered. As he spoke, the patient experienced overwhelming sadness. He was a very reserved and conservative man. We suggested that he continue his private thoughts during his manual physical therapy session. During that session, the anguish on his face was clear. We recommended a private place to cry and grieve. We respected his grief and chose not to pry because we were not invited. The following week, the patient said, "I think I was left with the memory of the pain. I feel much better now. My face doesn't hurt."

DISCUSSION

It is always important to work closely with the patient, to be open-minded, and to ask the patient what he/she remembers or feels is related to the injury.

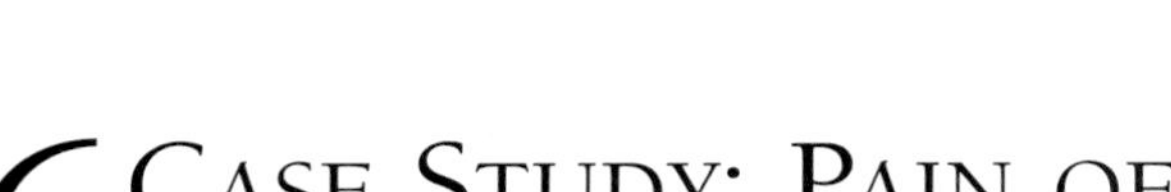

6 Case Study: Pain of Coccygeal Origin

HISTORY

A 20-year-old college student was referred by a physical therapy student. The history revealed that at age 14, the patient had fallen on her coccyx (tailbone) when one of her classmates pulled a chair out from under her. A few months after the incident, the patient began to experience low back pain along with headaches and neck pain. The parents sought conventional medical treatment. The patient saw numerous consultants, including the family physician, orthopedic surgeons, and chiropractors. The parents then took their daughter across the country to an osteopathic physician. He tried homeopathic techniques, including energy-field work, to relieve her pain. The patient also had extensive manual manipulation and high-velocity manipulation. As the years progressed, she did experience intermittent pain relief. During the last pain episode, the patient experienced excruciating, intractable pain in the coccygeal area. She also had pain with bowel movements, during her menstrual cycle, and when she sat.

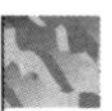

PERTINENT PHYSICAL FINDINGS

Evaluation of the patient's structure showed forward head carriage with anterior rotation of the shoulders and indentation of the upper chest. Her pelvis was tilted forward and twisted. The area over the coccyx was extremely sensitive to touch. X-rays of the coccyx were assessed by the radiologist as being within normal limits. However, when the x-rays were read in the office, it was noted that the coccyx was displaced toward the front.

TREATMENT

The treatment plan was discussed with the patient and her mother. The displaced coccyx was causing pain, and it made sense to reposition the coccyx into normal alignment. However, because of the pain, the patient could not tolerate manipulation of the coccyx. To numb the coccyx, the patient was given three caudal blocks with local anesthesia over the course of two weeks. At the end of this she was able to tolerate manual therapy. Aggressive manual techniques, including internal pelvic release, were used for direct manipulation of the coccyx. The patient also was able to tolerate extensive release of the iliopsoas muscles, which is normally very painful. At the end of six weeks of manual release physical therapy, the patient exited from our care essentially pain-free.

DISCUSSION

One of the most important aspects of the management of this patient was the sensory block, which provided not only complete temporary relief

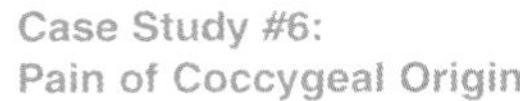

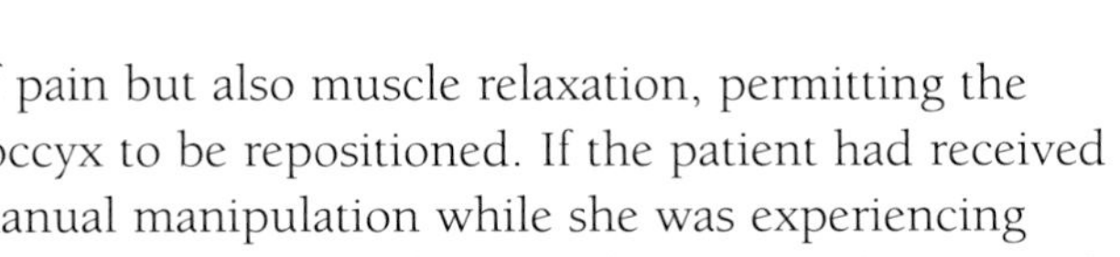

of pain but also muscle relaxation, permitting the coccyx to be repositioned. If the patient had received manual manipulation while she was experiencing extreme pain, natural body reflexes would have made realignment of the coccyx very difficult. It also would have taken twice as long to treat the problem.

8 Case Study: Arachnoiditis

HISTORY

A 27-year-old man was referred to the office by a prominent neurosurgeon for treatment of post-lumbar-laminectomy syndrome. The patient had had two previous lumbar laminectomy operations. The initial operation was performed six years prior to evaluation, and the second operation was performed one year prior to evaluation at Injury Specialists. The patient stated he had basically been well until two years before when he fell six feet off the back of an 18-wheel flatbed truck. At that time, he ripped the cartilage in his left knee and herniated a disc in his back, which was surgically removed. After the operation he had physical therapy, which included work-hardening (weight training, lifting, etc.). Subsequently, the patient experienced increased pain in his lower back radiating down the back of the left leg and excruciating pain in the left hip.

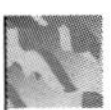

PERTINENT PHYSICAL FINDINGS

At the time of evaluation, the patient had pain while sitting, standing, lifting, and riding in a car; with weather changes, touch, and stress; and with defecation. His pain was relieved by changing positions and taking narcotic medications. His sleep was extremely disrupted. He was unable to work and unable to play with his young children.

The patient was 5'11" tall and weighed 300 pounds. Raising his left leg 30 degrees while he lay on his back created excruciating left hip and back pain. The patient could not bend over to touch the floor nor could he lean backwards or rotate to the right or left without pain in the hip. The most recent MRI of the lumbar spine showed a large mass pinching the spinal cord. This was consistent with the diagnosis of post-laminectomy syndrome, or arachnoiditis, meaning inflammation of the membrane that encloses the spinal cord.

TREATMENT

The treatment course for this patient included three lumbar epidural steroid injections, one week apart, and manual physical therapy. The patient failed to improve with this conservative regime, and his demands for narcotic medication increased. The recommendation was made for the patient to have a spinal cord stimulator implanted to treat the arachnoiditis syndrome. (The stimulator is an electrical device that short-circuits the nerve root signal, altering the pain sensation.) Approval for the spinal cord stimulator from the insurance company took approximately two months.

During this time, the patient developed a

narcotic addiction; he was taking almost 30 pills of codeine a day and was soliciting prescriptions from other physicians. After he missed several appointments, we confronted him, and he admitted to the narcotic addiction, stating that his pain was excruciating. He was also taking excessive Tylenol and multiple anti-inflammatory medications. We explained to the patient that he could suffer severe liver damage or renal failure from the excess medications. We pressured the insurance company to expedite approval of the spinal cord stimulator. Eventually, three months after the initial evaluation, the patient had a temporary spinal cord stimulator placed, which relieved the symptoms, then a permanent stimulator was implanted by a neurosurgeon. The patient was strong-willed and able to wean himself off the narcotics with the help of antidepressant medication.

DISCUSSION

The patient was able to detoxify himself from the narcotics, which is very difficult. He returned to our office walking briskly and stating that he was not taking any more medication and he was again able to enjoy life with his children. Overall, the patient had a very good result in spite of permanent nerve root scar damage.

9 Case Study: Wrist and Hand Pain

HISTORY

A 33-year-old man was referred by a nurse case manager for evaluation and treatment of wrist and hand pain. The patient, who was a laborer, was injured at work when he fell off a scaffold and fractured his right wrist. The day of the fracture he was seen in the emergency room and had the fracture appropriately treated. The emergency room physician referred the patient to an occupational therapist for rehabilitation after the cast was removed. The patient had approximately $7,000 worth of occupational therapy treatment, which was not helpful in relieving the pain. Eventually, the patient was referred to a hand surgeon who performed an EMG diagnostic test to evaluate nerve function. The EMG results were nonspecific but were consistent with an abnormality in the hand. Subsequently, one year after the original injury a hand surgeon performed a carpal tunnel release. The operation failed to relieve the pain, and the surgeon referred the patient to work-hardening physical therapy. One year later the patient developed worse wrist and hand pain from the physical therapy. He still had not been able to return to work. After the

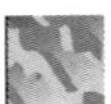

second round of physical therapy, the patient had repeat x-rays, a bone scan, and a wrist arthrogram study (x-ray dye study of a joint) in search of a diagnosis. The patient then saw two additional hand surgeons; one recommended fusing some of the wrist bones, the other recommended complete wrist fusion. Both hand surgeons stated clearly in their consultation notes that they did not know if the fusions would ease the patient's pain. Eventually, 18 months later, the patient was evaluated in our office.

PERTINENT PHYSICAL FINDINGS

The history revealed that the patient had wrist and hand pain with movement. The patient's forearm muscles were thoroughly palpated to evaluate for myofascial trigger points. The function of the wrist was evaluated completely. Flexion (bending) and supinating (rotating) the wrist caused pain. The patient's pain could be recreated by pressing the trigger points in the forearm muscles responsible for these movements.

TREATMENT

The patient was treated with three sessions of trigger point injections followed by manual physical therapy. At home the patient stretched his forearm muscles often.

DISCUSSION

Sadly, this case was misdiagnosed, and the social stress of the injury contributed to family problems and divorce. At the end of his treatment, the patient was told by the nurse case manager that his employer would not take him back. Fortunately, it was explained to the employer the patient was reliable and not malingering, and eventually he went back to work for the same company.

10 Case Study: Foot Pain

HISTORY

A 54-year-old waitress was referred for evaluation and treatment of right foot pain caused by a fall at work. Because of persistent foot and ankle pain, several diagnostic studies were ordered, including two MRIs, EMG, bone scan, and x-rays. Although the studies showed no abnormalities, an orthopedic surgeon made an incision on the top of the foot to release an entrapped nerve. The patient continued to have intense foot and ankle pain. Six months later we were asked to re-evaluate the patient. During the interview the patient was extremely agitated. She explained that when she slipped, all her weight had landed on the twisted ankle. The patient stated that she was told she might have sympathetically maintained pain. She was taking two antidepressants, two sedatives, one anti-inflammatory, and one muscle relaxant medication.

PERTINENT PHYSICAL FINDINGS

Physical examination revealed some hypersensitivity to touch. The patient walked favoring her

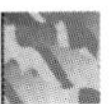

right leg. Because of chronic disuse, the muscles of the lower extremity were contracted. This trapped the blood and made her foot blue and swollen. The patient had significant palpable trigger bands in several of the lower leg muscles, which referred pain straight to the foot.

TREATMENT

The patient was treated for approximately six weeks with four sessions of trigger point injections to the calf muscles and myofascial release physical therapy. At the end of her treatment, she walked normally and was pain-free.

DISCUSSION

During the course of her treatment, the patient was weaned off all medications except one anti-depressant. With the therapy and medication changes, she became calm and focused. At the end of the treatment, she was able to walk well and stated she felt great. The patient exited from our care, saying, "You know, Doc, I used to think you were crazy, but now I have proof that you are anything but."

11 Case Study: Craniosacral Therapy

HISTORY

A 21-year-old woman was referred by a neurosurgeon for treatment of neck, head, and shoulder pain sustained in a major automobile accident three years earlier. The patient said she also experienced "rushes" of increased heart rate and sweating which were not related to agitation. Her history was complicated; she had fractured her neck and undergone fusion of five neck vertebrae.

PERTINENT PHYSICAL FINDINGS

Distortion of her face and skull were obvious: her eyes were not even, the cheekbone on the right was higher than on the left, and the left side of her face appeared depressed. Her right shoulder was higher than the left. She had a thick six-inch scar on the back of her neck from the operation. Because of the fusion she had a 50% decrease in neck range of motion. She walked bent forward and had a torsion

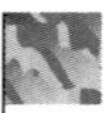

in the pelvis. There were multiple rotations in the thoracic spine.

TREATMENT

As we treated this patient with trigger point injections and manual therapy, her pain level decreased and her sleep pattern normalized, but her "rushes" did not improve. One month after completing her treatment, we saw her for a follow-up visit to make sure she continued to stay well. In spite of therapy, her previously corrected structural patterns had slipped back to abnormal positions. It became clear she had a cranial lesion. We referred her to a gifted osteopathic physician who specializes in cranial movement. After three weeks of craniosacral treatment, the "rushes" were gone, the patient had less pain and felt more vital, and her face returned to normal.

DISCUSSION

At that time our rehabilitation team did not feel proficient to treat cranial lesions. Because of this case, we have ongoing continuing education in this field and treat cranial lesions as indicated.